Hope for the Future

A Career Development Guide for Physician Executives

by Barbara J. Linney, MA

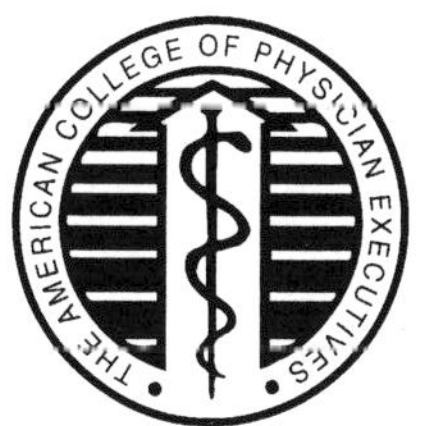

The American College of Physician Executives
4890 West Kennedy Boulevard, Suite 200
Tampa, Florida 33609-2575
813/287-2000

ISBN: 0-924674-47-4

Library of Congress Card Number: 96-086461

Printed in the United States of America by Hillsboro Printing, Tampa, Florida.

Preface

I have a theory, warmed by experience even though unsubstantiated by hard evidence, that almost every physician now plowing the management fields will find him- or herself unemployed at least once in the years ahead. Just as likely, I think, each physician executive will find it necessary to reinvent him- or herself and locate new opportunities in a health care field that is under constant change.

The race in all this will go to the swift and the flexible—to those who can anticipate changes in the structure and hiring needs of the health care field and respond to them aggressively. Those wedded to the status quo will find it difficult to survive in medicine and impossible to survive in medical management. Even many swift and flexible souls will struggle in an environment characterized by intense competition. Health care organizations will be battling for customers, and their managers will be asked on a regular basis to show what they've done for the organization lately.

But there will continue to be places for persons who can operate at the edge of the marriage between medicine and management. It is unlikely that the purpose of health care, the entrepreneurial noises of some notwithstanding, will ever be other than the provision of health care services. And the person who understands the nuances of health care delivery can expect a place, a significant place, in the health care delivery world.

That place will have to be won, however; it will not be given. This book, I think, shows how to prosper if your chosen profession is medical management. There are reasons for optimism, but there are also reasons to prepare for the very different employment world ahead.

Roger Schenke
Executive Vice President
American College of Physician Executives
October 1996

Introduction

The following quote was in a book called *Crisis Proof Your Career.* "'This is a test....This is only a test. Had this been your real life, you would have been shown where to go and what to do."[1] This sarcastic jolt reminds us—this is my one and only life, and I won't be given a set of instructions. I have to figure out what I want to do. Effective, happy people make those decisions for themselves, but it takes time. You must sit still, be reflective, figure out what you want and how to get it. No process guarantees that you will get everything you want, but many have reported that they feel a sense of meaning in their lives, some direction from a higher power, when they have taken the time to reflect and plan. "The goal...is to create...a plan—one that is loose enough for providence to intervene and tight enough to keep...on course month by month."[2]

In these turbulent times for health care, we wanted in this book to offer hope for your future and guide you in making career plans for yourself whether you move toward medical management, stay in clinical practice, or leave medicine altogether.

Chapter 1 describes the types of physician executive jobs people in the know are predicting for the future. Chapters 2, 3, and 4 will help you examine your professional and personal lives and prepare for change. Chapter 5 discusses how to get the experience that organizations and recruiters want you to have. Chapter 6 discusses communication skills needed for success. Chapters 7, 8, and 9 describe the "get down and dirty" skills of getting a job—networking, resumes, and interviews. Chapter 10 has advice for negotiating salaries. Chapter 11 tells how to cope with getting fired. Finally, Chapter 12 suggests some tools to use throughout the job search process.

Viktor Frankl wrote in *Man's Search for Meaning,* "Life ultimately means taking the responsibility to find the right answer to its problems and to fulfill the tasks which it constantly sets for each individual." I hope that you will find some of the answers you need in this book and that you will move in the direction you want to go.

References

1. Marion, P. *Crisis Proof Your Career.* New York, N.Y.: Berkley Books, 1994, p. 128.

2. *Ibid.* p. 129.

3. Frankl, V. *Man's Search for Meaning.* New York, N.Y.: Washington Square Press, 1985, p.98.

About the Author

Barbara J. Linney is Director of Career Development for the American College of Physician Executives. She is recognized nationally for her work in career counseling, management development, and communications training. Barbara's successful background includes one-on-one counseling in organizational and interpersonal skills, seminar presentations, articles published in health care and management periodicals, and college-level teaching.

Ms. Linney is a graduate of Westhampton College, Richmond, Virginia; earned her master's degree from the University of North Carolina-Charlotte; and has completed coursework for a doctorate from the University of South Florida, Tampa.

Contents

Chapter One

What Jobs Will Be There in the Future?

Physicians often ask me what kinds of jobs there will be for physician executives in the future. Lowell Weiner, MD, says, "...the demand for trained physician managers is greater than ever and increasing. The source of that demand is largely based on the needs of organizations that deliver or pay for health care. The demand increases as more of these organizations become involved in managed care in one form or another."[1]

I have interviewed two futurists and three recruiters to get their opinions about what physician executives will be doing. There is no universal agreement on exactly what the jobs will entail, but all agreed that physician executives will be needed. Several of the people speak of the traditional role of the medical director, so I'll list the tasks that have often been done by them. I compiled this list after reading many job descriptions. No one person would do all of them.

- Direct utilization review.
- Oversee quality assurance.
- Recruit physicians.
- Evaluate physician performance.
- Manage physician performance.
- Manage impaired physicians.
- Serve as liaison between administration and medical staff.
- Oversee credentialing and privileging of physicians.
- Develop provider relations.
- Resolve grievances.
- Mediate professional disputes and interdepartmental problems.
- Serve on board of directors.
- Develop staffing plans.

- Prepare expense budget for medical department.
- Ensure compliance with the mission statement, corporate policies, and bylaws.
- Participate in strategic planning.
- Ensure that medical staff efforts meet or exceed standards of various accrediting and approving bodies.[2]

The Futurists

Russell Coile Jr., President, Health Forecasting Group, Santa Clarita, California

Coile describes six types of jobs that will require physician executives and also made some predictions about which way the political winds are blowing in Washington.

There will continue to be a need for physician executives because, as organizations continue to cut costs, physician executives will be needed to be sure the quality of patient care is protected and to use their business acumen to reduce costs, thus helping the organization survive.

When the dust settles, physicians are likely to be working at five or six different major kinds of occupations around health care systems. I expect that VPMAs will have job titles such as vice president for clinical affairs and will be in charge of medical care. These will be the doctors who run the medical side of organizations. Managing physician performance will be the essence of the job.

The second type job would be an outcomes research job that's more scientific. The physician executive would be gathering information and doing clinical studies around best medical practices and new technology. He or she would head up a large research organization probably in a multihospital system and HMO.

A third possibility is that we will see physicians become the chief operating officers of hospitals and health systems because they have a strong clinical background. They will be managing the clinical side of the system and will deal with patient care operations—oversee nurses, techs, everybody.

A fourth job title would be physicians' becoming CEOs. A number of larger hospitals, particularly large academic medical centers, have historically had physicians as CEOs. This trend will spread to other types of organizations.

The fifth role, HMO medical director, is going to be a very important responsibility. There is already a significant number of HMO medical directors, so this is not a new career path, but as managed care comes to dominate the total American health care marketplace, these are going to be strategically significant positions. The physician will probably be the number two or three person in the

HMO. Above him or her would be the CEO. These plans are going to have millions of enrollees.

The window of opportunity for becoming an HMO medical director is the next 5-10 years. Last year, 46 new HMOs were started—half of them by providers. Not only will there be regional medical directors at the national level, but also each market will have its own medical director. If you have a multistate HMO that is operating in 10 states, each of those states will have its own medical director.

A sixth role for physicians is in sales and marketing for pharmaceutical firms, device makers, and medical technology companies. These companies are cutting back sharply on nonclinical marketing staff. They will expand the physician component. The pharmaceutical manufacturers and device makers will take a sales and marketing team to major corporate clients. That major corporate client may be an HMO, an organization such as Columbia HCA, a regional delivery system, or a regional or national group purchasing organization. The lead member of that team will be a physician. Pharmaceuticals and devices of the future are going to be sold on the basis of a combination of cost factors and clinical performance. The nonclinical marketing staff is going to be useless in that environment. They don't know the core business of patient care.

The pharmaceutical industries will look for two kinds of physicians to fill these positions in sales and marketing. One set of physicians will be young researchers who really know the science. The second will be a new set of physicians who are entrepreneurial and have a sales orientation.

There will definitely be a demand for physician executives in the future. As a theme under managed care and capitation, managing patient care will be the core business of health care enterprises, so we are going to need a lot of physician executive leadership. The blurring of the boundaries between the clinical side and the business side is occurring very rapidly, and the point at which the blurring happens is around the physician executive.

Leland Kaiser, President, Kaiser and Associates, Brighton, Colorado

I think there is going to be a progression in careers from physician to physician executive to physician community developer. There are going to be all kinds of jobs available in the future for doctors who work in communities to try to improve habitats to reduce the amount of disease in the population. Not like the old public healthers, but they will incorporate that knowledge. The future of health care is habitat redesign. You can't be healthy if you live in an unhealthy habitat. What we've always done is say we're not going to look at the habitat. We'll just look at people when they come to the emergency department. Now we are saying, "Let's get the lead paint off the walls so they don't come in the emergency department." That will be a whole employment sector.

Capitated managed care plans will pay for this examination of the community. They are going to enroll a whole population of people, do home visits, and then take a look at the factors in that neighborhood that are influencing the health of the people they are insuring. The idea is that if we can keep them out of the emergency department and keep them from calling doctors, we are going to make a lot of money in the process. Physician executives will be employed by the insurance plan.

The insurance plan may be a part of a hospital and a medical staff—some kind of corporate structure that brings together doctors, hospitals, and insurance plans under one umbrella. That's what I'd guess. So it will not be a pure insurance plan, but a new integrated delivery system that insures a population and is working with its own hospital and its own doctors, and some of those doctors will be specialized in the community.

A second tremendous use of physician executives will be teaching allopathic physicians how to work with complementary and alternative practitioners—herbalists, homeopaths, naturopaths, massage therapists, biofeedback, experts in acupuncture and acupressure, rolfing therapists—on down a long list. The reason is that there is good evidence to suggest we could probably reduce health insurance premiums 10 or 15 percent by using alternative and complementary medicine appropriately. The kicker in all this is that all the doctors that are currently out there have not been trained in alternative medicine. Many of the medical schools are now teaching those courses. There will be an integrated medical clinic—family-centered, neighborhood-based, one medical record—and it will integrate 20 or 30 alternative practitioners with regular physicians. Its idea will be, "We'll do what is appropriate here."

A third new employment place for physicians will be what I call potentiation. When I take a look at the evolution of medical care, it goes through three distinct stages: the treatment stage; the prevention and life styling stage, which we have just discussed a little bit; and then the potentiation stage, where what physicians are going to be doing is working to help people achieve their full 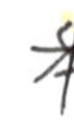 potential—physically, emotionally, mentally, and spiritually. So potentiation goes way beyond wellness. A good example would be that the many people whom we now call frail elderly wouldn't be frail if they used their muscles. And many elderly people who have brain dysfunctions of one type or another wouldn't if they still used their minds. Another good example would be that the kind of people we put in nursing homes in America are out doing Thai Chi exercises in China.

So there is a whole place here for a doctor now to begin to say, "How much physical potential is in your body that you've never used?" A physician will oversee this with other extenders. The physicians of the future are always going to work as a team. There are no solo actors in the future. The team will end up doing a profile on the person. They will look at unused potential. This could be a very sick person or a very healthy person. What you are asking is, How much unutilized potential is there. In addition to paying attention to their physical capabilities, we will ask how can we help them feel more, be more compassionate, be more loving—the whole emotional spectrum. How do we get their minds to work better—better memory, better analytic ability. Spirit—how can we help them achieve some greater sense of meaning and participation in the universe. Theoretically, my definition of a healthy person is simply a person who has achieved all of his or her potential in those four areas. Those are some of the new things we are going to be doing.

Then there is what I call the high-tech physician. This will be the physician manager who is really looking at things like nanotechnology, microrobotics, quantum medicine, genetic engineering. A whole high-tech end that is coming very quickly. The question here is, How do we use these high tech services? How do we pay for them? How do we organize them? How do we staff them? It is going to be a whole new arena, and, by the middle of the next century, all medical care will be driven by technology. We will have body scanners. What a patient will do is just come in and stand there, and there will be an atomic scan that will be fed into a computer that will do the diagnosis and then spit out some kind of a program to help the individual. Physicians will be programming the scanners and working with them so that each time they learn something new it is put into the scanner. Of course, there will always be a place for human judgment. As smart as the machines get, they are not living things. The physician has intuition. It's pretty hard to build intuition into a computer.

Will the physician still be the person who is offering human touch? Yes, although I must say that, once we move into the healing dimension, which is coming very quickly, there are many people in addition to physicians who will be doing that, and some of the physicians won't because they are just not healing people to begin with. So we'll make another distinction, along three areas: physicians who are more technologically oriented, those who are really more management oriented, and those who are more healing oriented. Nurses are doing most of the healing now, because nurses have a much more holistic attitude toward patients than doctors do.

One other thing. My belief is that health policy and health legislation should be drawn up by physicians. I don't know how much of a job category it's going to be because it's too early to tell. Physicians are not currently involved in this legislation. There is a whole new arena in what I call politics, policy science that says that, once doctors have had experience as clinicians, as managers, as technicians, all that kind of stuff, they will probably know enough to be trusted the first time to do policy. Now, a 35-year-old, newly admitted MBA is doing it. That's why we are in so much trouble. I think there will be a political dimension that will develop, but how big it will be I don't know at this time.

I think we are going to demand that our laws be drafted by experts but be reviewed and voted in by what I call the common person. I don't think experts ought to have the power to make laws. I think they should have the power to draft laws. Now, a lot of drafting is done by people that I don't think have the expertise to do it. I'd like to see a group of physicians who specialize in political action, in politics, and medicine and who draw what they feel would be the very best policies we could use but also have other people who are nonphysicians, the general populist type, review the policies and finally either vote them in or vote them down. Now what happens is just the results of politics, and you don't have the science in there. I think as we move in the future we are not going to let it be that sloppy.

My guess is that, in the next century, we are going to have a self-designing America and that educational levels are going up with the Internet and the information society. People are finally going to get to the point that they can intelligently review how policy is made. At that point, we are going to have a downward delegation of powers from the federal and state governments to the local level. It is already happening in Canada. Local citizens will be much more involved in running their schools, their welfare programs, their health programs, and so forth. So the federal government is going to let go of some of the money and power to revitalize our democracy. This creates a role for people, such as physicians, to get involved at the local level.

The Recruiters

Jennifer Grebenschikoff, Vice President, Physician Executive Management Center, Tampa, Florida

We are seeing a move away from the traditional medical director job. Even the traditional VPMA is only spending 10-15 percent of his or her time on traditional responsibilities. A physician still needs to handle things such as credentialing, physician discipline, and medical staff issues, but we are seeing these physicians hiring very competent medical staff coordinators to handle by-laws, meetings, getting ready for the Joint Commission, and all those sorts of things. Whereas before you had a medical staff secretary who sent the meeting notices out, now you have medical staff coordinators who are assuming much more responsibility in that area. So the VPMA is freed up to do other things.

We cannot present candidates who don't have skills in performance improvement, which is the whole issue of clinical pathways, guidelines, disease state management processes—the things you need to use and do to help physicians look at their practice patterns and change them to be able to survive in a capitated world. I use the word capitated instead of managed care because a lot of physicians think discounted fee for service is managed care, and it is not. Capitation is taking risks. Employers also want physicians who have had significant experience in settings where the organization has relied on its revenues from capitation, not just a discounted fee for service. There are many good physicians who have done it.

Organizations that have never had a physician executive before are looking around and saying, we have this wonderful management team, but we don't have a physician component on it, so we are not seeing any decrease in demand for physician executives. Even when physicians say their positions were eliminated, it is not that the position was truly eliminated; their slot was eliminated because of a merger. The position itself is still valuable to organizations. If you have two 250-bed hospitals that merge, you don't need two VPMAs. We are seeing more and more organizations waking up and saying, How can we possibly build physician networks and integrate our physicians into our system if we don't have a strong physician executive to help us?

Our clients also want physicians who have dealt with clinical information systems and have used those data to help physicians look at their practices, who are analyzing which electronic medical record to use, who are figuring out how to get PCs on the desk of every physician and to show them how to use hand-held computers. Before, all that was done through the medical records department. Now the physician executive works closely with information services staff or the chief information officer. However, it has to be a large organization before it can afford to have the physician executive serve as the chief information officer (CIO).

Management education will be important. There are beginning to be so many people with management degrees that you start to lose a bit of an edge if you don't have one. Clients are still looking for whether this person has made a commitment to management through continuing education or an advanced degree. So for the future, you have to take courses and go to school.

Sue Cejka, President, Cejka & Company, St. Louis, Missouri

In major metropolitan areas, in sophisticated health systems, I think the role of the medical director will probably head toward a person in charge of informatics, outcomes, clinical pathways. In single hospitals in nonmetropolitan areas, I think the role will remain traditional.

In many respects, managed care is grossly overstated. I had lunch today with the president of a health plan in St. Louis. He came out of California, so he really knows global capitation. They've got about 60,000 enrollees in the St. Louis market. They pay all their doctors on a discounted fee-for-service basis. All the hype we hear about managed care and about HMOs is not necessarily factual. Fundamentally, life does not change until you have to live with capitation. A 4,000-bed hospital system is recruiting a medical director, but in my opinion they want a traditional medical director. They would tell you otherwise, but, if I really look behind the job, I'm going to tell you it is a traditional medical director. I think this is changing, but it is changing much more slowly than any of the media have really acknowledged.

Arkansas just passed an all-payer law. Any doctor who is willing to accept the fee schedule given by the payer is eligible. You can't select out on the basis of quality, outcomes, or clinical pathways. Even the job of the traditional medical director will be changed in places where this law is passed, and about 10 states have passed that legislation. The medical director's hands will be tied if he or she can't select qualified physicians on the basis of quality, outcomes, or clinical pathways. The credentialing process will be paralyzed.

John Lloyd, Witt/Kieffer, Ford, Hadelman & Lloyd, Oak Brook, Illinois

I have seen no physician executives downsized out of positions without plenty of lead time and plenty of leeway. When three big systems combined, they ended up with three medical directors. One kept the title of Senior Vice President of Medical Affairs. One took the title of Vice President of Medical Education and was satisfied with the position. The other one took the title of Vice President of Physician Outreach and did it for about six months. It was not the job he wanted. He decided to move, and they provided him a good bit of severance in the process.

The positions are being altered and merged, but not eliminated. Organizations still want medical directors. Here is a list of qualifications that organizations are telling us they want in the executives whom they are hiring. A successful executive:

- Has a vision and understands on a broad perspective where health care is and where it is going.
- Can clearly articulate that vision and can lead people to it. The communication skills of the executive are more critical today than at any time in the past 25 years.
- Has ego—not egotistical—strength, because you are not going to be loved by all. The chances are you are going to be loved by few.
- Has the ability to manage change. It is not going to be the way it was before.
- Is able and willing to select excellent talent and not be intimidated by having that talent ready to solve problems. There is not an executive in this country who can do it all.
- Knows how to use information. You don't have to be completely computer literate, but you must know what to do with computer-generated information.
- Is fair; is demanding but has an understanding and a reason to be patient with people in trying to help the whole group move forward.
- Has appropriate background and title before coming to us.

◆ ◆ ◆ ◆

Some of these experts see the medical director position becoming more specialized. Others see it continuing with the traditional tasks of managing physician behavior, overseeing utilization review and quality assurance, paying attention to budgets. Whatever they are doing, Lowell Weiner, MD, says they will be needed in the future: "[T]he demand for trained physician managers is greater than ever and increasing. The source of that demand is largely based on the needs of organizations that deliver or pay for health care. The demand increases as more of these organizations become involved in managed care in one form or another."[1]

Many experts agree the window of opportunity of demand for physician executives is the next 5 to 10 years. This book is meant to help you be ready to take advantage of that opportunity. Organizations want a person with management experience, excellent communication skills, and a flexible attitude, and a person willing to learn whatever skills are needed to handle the changes that are here and the many that will surely come. The remaining chapters will help you examine what you are doing now, what has led you to this point in your life, what you want to do next, and how you can be a desirable candidate to fill a physician executive position.

References

1. Weiner, L. "The Transition from Clinician to Manager." In *Physicians in Managed Care.* Bloomberg, M., and Mohlie, S., Editors. Tampa, Fla.: American College of Physician Executives, 1994, p. 46.

2. Linney, G., and Linney, B. *Medical Directors: What, Why, How.* Tampa, Fla.: American College of Physician Executives, 1992, p. 3.

Chapter Two

Life-Work Planning Can Give You Energy

Having read about the types of jobs that people in the know predict will exist in the future, I'd like you to back away from the specifics of the profession and take a careful look at your own career thus far. What are the characteristics of your work experience and your personal life? The assessment of these areas is the first step in a process commonly referred to as Life-Work Planning.

The term implies that you can plan your life and your work and not just let events happen to you. You plan and then relax—not holding onto the plan too tightly. Most things I've wanted desperately have come to me after I let up from desperately wanting them. I turned my attention to something else, and then what I desired seemed to just come and sit in my lap. But this does not mean that you passively wait. You set goals, write them down, and then do activities that work toward the goals and that can make you enjoy life's journey.

In order to plan your future, it is a good idea to take time to assess your career—think about the present, take a look back at your past, and then look toward the future with a plan of action. I am going to discuss ways to examine your present with the help of some writing exercises and an overview of an instrument that measures your likes and dislikes. Writing is an excellent way to examine your life. It can enable you to do life-work planning on your own.

Begin by making a list of energizers and deenergizers. Use the work sheets at the end of the chapter. (Such work sheets will appear in most of the chapters so that you can become involved with the techniques prescribed in this book immediately.) Energizers are activities or people that excite you. You have more energy after doing them or being with them than you did when you began. Deenergizers are activities or people who drain you of energy quickly. You feel tired and maybe even depressed after a short time.

Examples of Energizers

My List

- Speaking to a large group
- One-on-one educational coaching sessions
- Long walks
- Talk with a good friend
- Dancing
- Writing

One Physician's List

- Helping colleagues or patients solve problems
- Completing tasks in a timely manner
- Talking with a good friend
- Serious exercise or competitive sports

Examples of Deenergizers

My List

- Continuous conflict
- Trying to work when there is a lot of noise
- Filing papers
- Parties with large numbers of people
- Preparing income tax records

A Physician's List

- Long and/or disorganized meetings
- Confronting a fellow physician about something unpleasant
- Budget preparation

After you've made these lists, I suggest filling out a personality instrument called the Myers-Briggs Type Indicator to help you further understand why you like some activities and don't like others. It reinforces for you why some things turn you on and others turn you off.

To find out who gives the test in your area, contact the headquarters of the Association for Psychological Type, 816/444-3500, and ask it for an APT chapter in your area. We give the test in the ACPE Career Choices program and in One-on-One Coaching sessions in Tampa.

It's important to know what your natural tendencies are when you are making career changes. I have heard physicians say that they are living a life that a 10-year-old boy or girl chose for them. Many were that young when they made the decision to become doctors. One obstetrician told me he wished he had filled out the instrument in high school. He would never have chosen his specialty, obstetrics/gynecology, if he had known how much time alone he needed and how much interruptions bothered him.

The Myers-Briggs Type Indicator is based on Carl Jung's works. Jung, a Swiss psychiatrist (1875-1961) "believed we are born with a predisposition to certain personality preferences."[1] He came up with four sets of behaviors to describe how people usually behave. Katherine Briggs had been devising her own classification of personality differences when she read Jung and realized their theories were similar, but his were more thoroughly developed. "In 1942, prompted by World War II...and the conviction that the war was caused, in part, by people not understanding differences," Katherine Briggs and her daughter, Isabel Myers, "began to develop a series of questions to measure personality differences. The result was the Myers-Briggs Type Indicator."[2]

I'm going to briefly describe the behaviors in hopes that you will be able to say, "Yes, I'm somewhat like that one but not like that one," and then perhaps you will want to pursue the information further. The four sets of behaviors are:

Extrovert ....Introvert

Sensing.....................Intuitive

Thinking ....Feeling

Judging.....................Perceiving

The sets of behaviors describe our source of energy, how we take in information from the world, how we make decisions, and how we organize our lives. As you are deciding which behavior you prefer, keep in mind that everyone exhibits all eight behaviors, but most people in the population have at least a slight preference for one behavior in each of the sets.

The first sets (Extrovert and Introvert) explain our source of energy. (Try to forget society's definition of these two words—outgoing and shy. Jung used them differently.) Extroverts get energy from people and from activities outside themselves. They want to talk to others a lot, often working out their thoughts aloud as they talk. Introverts get energy from within themselves. They usually need a fair amount of time alone and prefer to do their thinking quietly to themselves and then let others know what they have worked out.

Extroverts begin to talk and then, seven or eight sentences later, they know what they really think. Introverts often think extroverts have lied to them at the beginning of the conversation, but it's not necessarily so. They are just working through a problem out loud while the introvert would do all the thinking internally and then deliver the finished product.

Similarly, extroverts can be annoyed with introverts because they resent that introverts didn't let them in on any of their quiet thinking process.

"If you don't know what an Extrovert is thinking...you haven't been listening, because he or she will tell you. If you don't know what an Introvert is thinking...you haven't asked, or, in some cases, you haven't waited long enough for an answer....Introverts 'bake' their ideas inside, much as cake is cooked in the oven and presented to the outside world only after it is finished."[3]

Kroeger and Thuesen write, "If you are an Extrovert, you tend to talk first, think later, and don't know what you'll say until you hear yourself say it....You probably know a lot of people and count many of them among your 'close friends'....If you are an Introvert, you probably rehearse things before saying them and prefer that others would do the same....You like to share special occasions with just one other person or perhaps a few close friends."[4]

At work, extroverts like variety and action. They like to have lots of people around in the working environment. Introverts at work like quiet for concentration, and they can work alone contentedly for long periods.

Physician executives who are extroverts probably enjoy most the part of the job that requires that they speak to groups or walk around the medical facility talking with co-workers. Introverts may be most comfortable managing information or doing quality assurance and utilization review.

"About 75 percent of the American population is Extroverted....If you are having trouble deciding which you prefer, ask yourself this question: 'If I had to be one way or the other for the rest of my life, which would I choose?'"[5]

Before you read about the next set of behaviors, write the answers to the following questions on the work sheets at the end of the chapter:

- Which term seems to describe how you like to do things, Extrovert or Introvert? Give one reason why.
- Is your life structured so you can do enough of this behavior to satisfy you? If so, how? If not, what could you change?

The second set of behaviors (Sensing and Intuitive) describe how we take in information about our world. Sensing types take in information through their five senses (sight, sound, smell, taste, and touch). Intuitives take in information through almost a sixth sense or a hunch. They think they know something, are not sure why, but are right often enough that they come to trust their hunches.

Sensing types like to work with details, and they approach projects in a step-by-step manner, starting at the beginning and proceeding until they are finished. They like established ways of doing things. These people often like to be involved with finance or technology and are very comfortable with numbers, computers, detailed procedures, etc. Because they don't mind repetition, their motto might be, "If it isn't broken, don't fix it."

Whereas sensing types are very comfortable with proven methods, intuitives rarely like to do the same thing twice. Their motto might be the same as that of a recent management book: *If It Ain't Broken, Break It.*[6] They like to start big projects, sometimes tackling the middle section first and skipping around from one idea to the next without a particular order. Intuitives see the big picture. They are often looking toward the future and imagining possibilities.

Intuitives often like executive positions where they are responsible for strategic planning or are called upon to solve unexpected problems. They often serve in counselor roles no matter what titles they have because they enjoy helping people think of possible changes they might make in their lives.

If you show a peanut to sensing types, they see a small brown object that is rough and appears to be two ball shapes joined together. Show it to intuitives and their first response might be, "Jimmy Carter raised peanuts." They will think of something beyond what they are actually looking at. These two types often annoy each other because of their different styles, but if they can work together without driving each other crazy, good things happen. Intuitives start some great projects and sensing types help them finish them, tending to many of the details. Each needs the other.

"If you are a Sensor, you probably prefer specific answers to questions; when you ask someone the time, you prefer 'three fifty-two' and get irritated if the answer is 'a little before four' or almost time to go....If you are an intuitive, you probably would rather fantasize about spending your next paycheck than sit and balance your checkbook."[7]

Sensors focus on "what is," while intuitives focus on "what could be." "About 75 percent of the American population are Sensors."[8]

Before you read about the next set of behaviors, write the answers to the following questions on the work sheets:

- Which term seems to describe how you like to do things, Sensing or Intuitive? Give one reason why.
- Is your life structured so you can do enough of this behavior to satisfy you? If so, how? If not, what could you change?

Once you've taken in information from your world, it's usually necessary to make decisions about it. The two sets of behaviors (Thinking and Feeling) explain how people prefer to make decisions. Thinking types make decisions based on what is logical and reasonable. Feeling types consider how the decision will affect other people and themselves.

Thinking types are very good at analyzing business plans or problems. They are often firm and tough-minded and may hurt other people's feelings without knowing it. If it makes economical sense to fire someone, they can do it without agonizing over the decision.

Whereas thinking types decide with their heads, feeling types decide with their hearts. Feeling types can and do fire people when necessary, but they suffer when they have to do it because they worry about hurting people's feelings and about the hardship such actions will cause employees families. Feeling types are good at understanding people. They like harmony and are willing to work to make it happen. "When Thinkers and Feelers clash, more often than not the Feeler ends up hurt and angry, while the Thinker is confused about what went wrong."[9]

"If you are a Thinker, you probably think it's more important to be right than liked; you don't believe it is necessary to like people in order to be able to work with them and do a good job....If you are a Feeler, you probably put yourself in other people's moccasins; you are likely to be the one in a meeting who asks, 'How will this affect the people involved?'"[10]

It's important to remember that thinking types have deep feelings and that feeling types think logically. Jung and the Myers-Briggs Type Indicator refer to how people make decisions, not to their ability to think or feel.

"The American population is evenly split between Thinkers and Feelers. However, this is the only type dimension in which clear gender differences show up. About two thirds of men prefer thinking, and about two thirds of women prefer feeling."[11]

Before you read about the next set of behaviors, write the answers to the following questions on your work sheets:

- Which term seems to describe how you like to do things, Thinking or Feeling? Give one reason why.
- Is your life structured so you can do enough of this behavior to satisfy you? If so, how? If not, what could you change?

The final sets of behaviors (Judging and Perceiving) describe how you organize your life. Judging types like to make decisions and get things settled quickly. They like to have order and structure, giving them a sense that they have life under control. Perceiving types like to continue to take in more information and keep their options open. They like to take each experience as it comes, without the feeling of being tied down to a plan.

"If you are a Judger, you probably thrive on order; you have a special system for keeping things in the refrigerator and dish drainer, hangers in your closets, and pictures on your walls....If you are a Perceiver, you don't believe that 'neatness counts,' even though you would prefer to have things in order; what's important is creativity, spontaneity, and responsiveness."[12]

Physician executives who are judging types are usually comfortable making decisions quickly—saying yes or no to a certain medical procedure on the basis of cost and quality of care. Perceiving types probably prefer tasks such as gathering a great deal of information before a piece of medical equipment is purchased.

"Judgers tend to live in an orderly way and are happiest when their lives are structured and matters are settled....Perceivers like to live in a spontaneous way and are happiest when their lives are flexible....Judgers seek to regulate and control life....Perceivers seek to understand life rather than control it."[13]

"The American population is evenly split on this dimension: 50 percent are Judgers, and 50 percent are Perceivers."[14]

Write the answers to the following questions in your workbooks:

- Which term seems to describe how you like to do things, Judging or Perceiving? Give one reason why.
- Is your life structured so you can do enough of this behavior to satisfy you? If so, how? If not, what could you change?

Remember—everyone can do all these different behaviors, but your comfort zone will tend to be in one area or the other of each of the pairs.

If you can identify which type you are, you can more easily choose work that is satisfying to you. Also, if you decide which of these behaviors you prefer and structure your life so you get to do them, you will find you have more energy. Here is a list of activities that you can do that will meet the needs of your preferred type.

Extroverts—Plan activities to be with people.

Introverts—Plan to have time alone.

Sensing—Do something that lets you have control over details. Write computer programs. Have a detailed filing system. Plan an elaborate dinner.

Intuitive—Use your imagination to come up with new projects. Write them down. Try to carry out some of them.

Thinking—Write a financial plan. Run your own business.

Feeling—Get with a friend and talk about your feelings. Do something good for someone else.

Judging—Be the one who makes decisions. You probably will not be happy unless you have the final say on some issues.

Perceiving—Gather information and let others make some of the decisions. Have an unscheduled Saturday when you do whatever occurs to you all day long.

Know yourself. Choose which behavior fits you. Fill out the Myers-Briggs instrument some time to get a more accurate assessment. The information may help explain why some things energize you and others deenergize you.

Life-work planning may involve changing jobs, but it may not. If you decide what energizes you and what deenergizes you and accept that fact without condemning your inadequacies, you can add activities to your life that satisfy you. If you meet the needs of each of your behavior types, you'll have the energy not only to be productive in your present situation but to choose new challenges.

I have talked to many physicians over the past five years who were somewhat disturbed that they wanted to do something besides clinical practice. Frankly, they were bored and wanted new challenges. Their families and friends did not want to hear such comments and their general reaction was "You're a doctor. What more could you want?" The authors of *Do What You Are* explain this restlessness as a normal part of adult growth. "Based on our experience with our clients, we believe that mid-life marks the beginning of a new phase of type development. Unconsciously, we seek to round out our personalities and become more effective and capable....[H]aving reached the top of the proverbial hill, we may also reach some disturbing conclusions: first, that there may not be that much time left ahead, and, second, that there isn't much challenge in spending the remaining years exactly as we spent our earlier years."[15]

Bluestein conducted a survey of 230 physicians who changed from clinical practice to management in a managed care setting. He interpreted the transition to an alternative career as a first cousin of mid-life crisis rather than a mid-career change. He said of his own change, "One of the primary motivations to do something else was looking down the road 30 years and realizing that most of my time was going to be spent doing pretty much the same old thing."[16]

The marketplace has changed a great deal in the past few years. Some specialists are out of work and, in some managed care organizations, even primary care doctors have lost jobs, because one physician with the help of physician extenders can see more patients than they used to. The turnover of physician executives is high. My sources tell me that a physician executive now lasts about 2.7 years in one position. Whatever is causing you to think about making changes, try to stay calm and take the time to think about your life and work before you make decisions about what to do next.

References

1. Kroeger, O., and Thuesen, J. *Type Talk.* New York, N.Y.: Delacorte Press, 1988, p. 281.
2. *Ibid.*, p. 282.
3. Tieger, P., and Barron-Tieger, B. *Do What You Are.* Boston, Mass.: Little, Brown, and Company, 1995, p. 15.
4. Kroeger, O., and Thuesen, J., *op. cit.*, pp. 14-15.
5. Tieger, P., and Barron-Tieger, B., *op. cit.*, p. 17.
6. Kriegel, R., and Patler, L. *If It Ain't Broke, Break It.* New York, N.Y.: Warner Books, 1991.
7. Kroeger, O., and Thuesen, J., *op. cit.*, pp. 18-19.
8. Tieger, P., and Barron-Tieger, B., *op. cit.*, p. 21.
9. *Ibid.*, p. 23.
10. Kroeger, O., and Thuesen, J., *op. cit.*, p. 19.
11. Tieger, P., and Barron-Tieger, B., *op. cit.*, p. 24.
12. Kroeger, O., and Thuesen, J., *op. cit.*, p. 21.
13. Tieger, P., and Barron-Tieger, B., *op. cit.*, p. 25.
14. *Ibid.*, p. 29.
15. *Ibid.*, p. 86.
16. Bluestein, P. "Physicians in Transition." *Physician Executive* 21(12):16-24, Dec. 1995.

Other Readings

Keirsey, D., and Bates, M. *Please Understand Me.* Del Mar, Calif.: Prometheus Nemesis Book Company, 1984.

Myers, I., with Myers, P. *Gifts Differing.* Palo Alto, Calif.: Consulting Psychologists Press, Inc., 1980.

Work Sheets

At the end of many of the chapters in this book, we have provided space for you to undertake the exercises that have been recommended. We encourage you to take the time to fill them out. If, like my editor, you wince at the prospect of writing in a book, just make photocopies. The important thing is to record your thoughts on these important topics when the juices are running.

Energizers/Deenergizers

These are the things in my life that energize me:

1. ______
2. ______
3. ______
4. ______
5. ______
6. ______
7. ______
8. ______
9. ______
10. ______

These are the things in my life that deenergize me:

1. ______
2. ______
3. ______
4. ______
5. ______
6. ______
7. ______
8. ______
9. ______
10. ______

Behavior Sets

Extrovert/Introvert

1. Which term seems to describe how you like to do things, Extrovert or Introvert? Give one reason why

2. Is your life structured so you can do enough of this behavior to satisfy you? If so, how? If not, what could you change?

Sensing/Intuitive

1. Which term seems to describe how you like to do things, Sensing or Intuitive? Give one reason why.

2. Is your life structured so you can do enough of this behavior to satisfy you? If so, how? If not, what could you change?

Thinking/Feeling

1. Which term seems to describe how you like to do things, Thinking or Feeling? Give one reason why.

2. Is your life structured so you can do enough of this behavior to satisfy you? If so, how? If not, what could you change?

Judging/Perceiving

1. Which term seems to describe how you like to do things, Judging or Perceiving? Give one reason why.

2. Is your life structured so you can do enough of this behavior to satisfy you? If so, how? If not, what could you change?

Chapter Three

Know Where You've Been Before You Decide Where to Go

In order to plan your future, it is a good idea to take time to think about the present, to take a look back at the past, and then to look toward the future with a plan of action. In Chapter 2, I suggested the Myers-Briggs Type Indicator to examine how you like to do things in the present. Now let's examine the past and future. In this chapter, I'll suggest strategies for reviewing your past and planning your future. Several times I'll ask you to write lists and then reflect on them.

Richard Bolles, in *The Three Boxes of Life,* described a study that was done on patients at a New York City hospital to see what made some patients heal faster than others after the same type of surgery. The researchers discovered that fast healers were those who believed there was some meaning to everything that happened to them, even if that meaning was not evident at the time of going through the experience.[1]

Such an attitude toward life is also helpful when you are well and considering major changes in your life. Meaning is a word with a slippery definition. It's an individual concept. My meaning will be different from yours. That's fine. It's just important that we both find some meaning in our lives.

If you can look back over your life and see a pattern that makes some sense to you, you feel secure, like you are on the right track. "People who have a sense of purpose are those who can take any random experience that happens to them and put it into some kind of larger perspective."[2] When you have a sense of purpose, you are more likely to find the courage to try new things, take on the next challenge. Lee Kaiser says, "Life can be viewed as an unfoldment process. This happened and this happened. What would be the next unfoldment? What would be the next logical step that seems to grow out of the past?"[3]

For example, when I moved to Florida in 1983, I decided to work on a PhD in Tampa. I lived in Orlando, so that meant driving 100 miles each way every week, spending 1 or 2 nights away from my family. I did the trek for three years and finished all the course work. In the last summer session, I turned in my proposal for my dissertation, which my professor and I had been working on for three months. He said, "I hope you will do this study sometime." I said,

"Sometime! I thought this *was* my dissertation proposal." He said, "Well, I don't know if the committee will approve it." I walked out thinking, "How much longer can I jump through academic hoops?"

At the same time, my first consulting job with the American Management Association landed in my lap. The woman who was supposed to do it couldn't for personal reasons. My consulting career took off once I had worked for AMA, because it is very respected in the profession.

For several years I thought, "Why did I drive to Tampa for three years?" It all seemed such a waste. The answer that finally occurred to me was, "So I could learn to spend the night alone in a hotel and not be afraid." I do that all the time now, but the first time I did it I barely slept, because I was afraid. I didn't get what I thought I wanted, but while working toward it, I got something else that I wanted more. When I make sense of an unexpected turn in my life, I have more courage to try new things and am less likely to be thrown off or be unsettled by the next surprise. "Soren Kierkegaard wrote, 'Life can only be understood backward, but it must be lived forward.'"[4] When you have found some understanding about the past, you are more ready to move forward.

In the last chapter, I asked you to spend a considerable amount of time thinking about what you like to do and don't like to do. Now I'd like you to look back over the events of your past. The Howards, in *Exploring the Road Less Traveled*, said, "Most of us learn best, *really* learn, from our own experience—not simply from having things happen to us but from reflecting on what happens, both alone and in exchanges with others, so that the meaning of our experience becomes clear and we can make choices based on growing awareness rather than unchallenged assumptions."[5]

Reviewing Your Past

A way to reflect on what has happened to you is to do an exercise recommended by Ira Progoff in his Journal Workshops. List the steppingstones of your life—the significant events that have led you to where you are today.[6] Don't feel this has to be a definitive list or that it has to be in a correct order. Just quickly write the items as they occur to you. On another day, the list would be different.

Example of Steppingstones of a Physician

- Born 1943
- Decision to be a doctor 1956
- College 1961
- Medical School 1965
- Pediatric Residency 1969
- Married 1971

- Moved to Charlotte to begin practice 1972
- Children 1972 and 1975
- First full-time management position. CIGNA, Orlando 1983
- Began consulting business 1988

Make your own list, using the work sheets at the end of the chapter. The old adage, "Those who do not study history are doomed to repeat it," applies to your personal history as well. After you've made your list, think about the following questions, writing your answers on the work sheets at the end of the chapter. The answers here are meant only for guidance. This, like all the exercises in this book, is an intensely personal experience:

- **What was good?** *I'm glad I became a surgeon. I've loved being able to quickly fix many problems.*
- **What was bad?** Decision to invest money in so and so.
- **What do you wish you had done?** *I wish I had become a history professor instead of going to medical school.*
- **What do you wish you had not done?** *I wish I had not divorced my first wife. In my third marriage, I'm still dealing with the same problems. I might as well have stayed in the first one and worked them out.*
- **Do you see some meaning or a pattern that makes sense to you?** One person told me that, when he looked back at the past, he saw a pattern of leaving situations quickly when they became difficult (a marriage, a job). He wanted to not do that in this crisis. He wanted to take his time, think, move slower, sit with the pain a little longer, and perhaps make a better decision than some he had made in the past.
- **Do you see a natural progression?** A woman said she kept admiring men who were doing what she wanted to do. She realized she learned something from each of them, and now she is doing it.

Answer the questions above for your own list of steppingstones, using the appropriate work sheets at the end of the chapter.

Often, we just keep living life at a breakneck speed without pausing to see what we can learn from what we have done. It is often scary to slow down and process events, but the rewards can be great if you can sit with the uneasiness a little while. Progoff claims that, to think about "the past periods of our lives gives us access to the unlived possibilities of our existence which the future may still give us an opportunity to fulfill, albeit in a different form."[7] Howard Figler, in *The Complete Job-Search Handbook*, says looking back at what you have done even allows you to get paid what you should. "Your ability to communicate your worth is a function of your ability to recognize value in your own experience and see how it can be translated into new capabilities."[8]

Planning Your Future

After you have thought about your present life, what you like to do and what you don't, and looked back at what has led you to where you are today, you are ready to set some goals for your future. List all of the things you want in your professional and private lives. Let your imagination run wild.

When you make the list, you may think all sorts of strange messages from the past: "I don't deserve it; I never really wanted it anyway; what about the starving, dying people who can't have what they want?; You are getting too big for your britches." Either ignore or write the thoughts down, but keep on making the list. Barbara Sher, in *I Could Do Anything If I Only Knew What It Was,* says, "You can trust desire....There's a practicality in our longings that's beyond rational thought. Your desire will point you in the right direction better than any rules or well-meant advice."[9] Try to overcome the forces of resistance that keep you from thinking about what you really want in life. Write anything you desire, even if it is unreasonable, because no one else will know about it unless you choose to tell them.

Examples

- Continued happy marriage
- Financial security in retirement
- Fulfilling work
- Continued good health
- Able to resume competitive running
- Satisfying church life.
- Kids will become happy, productive adults
- Make some impact on health care delivery, cost, service

Make your own list on the work sheets. After you've made an exhaustive list, pick one item that you would like to think more about. Write the answers to the following questions about that item on the work sheets at the end of the chapter. Again, the answers here are meant only for guidance.

- **What do you want?** Get out of clinical practice and into management.
- **What will you have to pay (sacrifice) to get it?** "The notion that you can simultaneously have it all is an illusion. Choices, sacrifices, and trade-offs are realities of life.[10]

  I need some experience and education. I may have to take a position that pays less than I get now in order to get experience.

- **What might get in the way, be an obstacle to getting what you want?**

  I live in a small town. There are no major clinics or hospitals that have or want medical directors. I may have to move.

- **Can you picture yourself already having it?** Write a paragraph describing yourself already having what you want.

  I am a good Vice President of Medical Affairs. I talk to physicians and administrators and try to get each to be patient with the other, to learn the art of compromising. I can tell physicians when they need to change behavior or practice patterns.

- **What one thing could you do today that would move you toward your goal?** You need short-, mid-, and long-term goals. Do something now to get you on the way. If a long-range goal is to be out of patient care and working in managed care or health insurance in five years, a short-term goal would be to volunteer to chair the utilization review committee at the hospital so you can get the kind of experience that is valued by potential employers. If you want to be a Vice President of Medical Affairs, find out what it takes to become chief of your clinical department or to get on the executive committee of your hospital. People who choose the VPMA career path have usually been heavily involved in the hierarchy of one or more hospital medical staffs.

- **What don't you want to do anymore?** Sometimes, if you can't figure out what you want to do, start with what you don't want to do. If you don't want to take night call anymore, how might you stop it? Can you pay someone else to take it? Can you take home less money to get out of it? Can you get more partners so you do it less often? Can you share call with a large group in town? Can you get out of clinical medicine?

- **What are your "Evil Secrets?"** This question "may help you clarify what you really want. One key to discovering what you really like and love is to ask yourself what are the things you don't like to admit. 'I don't like to admit it, but I need to be the center of attention.' O.K., find a career path that will let you show off. 'I don't like to admit it, but I don't like dealing with other people.' OK, then devise a role that will let you make your contribution through things done in your office, such as intellectual creativity and true technical superiority. 'I don't like to admit it, but I really want to be rich.' Fine, go out and build a business. 'I don't like to admit it, but I'm an intellectual snob.' That's all right, so find a career path that will allow you to work only with smart people. Play to your 'evil secrets.' Don't suppress them. You are a lot less flexible than you think."[11]

After you go through this exercise, you might want to explore in depth some other items from your want list by using the above questions. Extra work sheets are provided for expanding this exercise. When you've thought about it as much as you want to, make a list of the top three to five items you want to keep in mind. Several years ago, an insurance company in Hartford, Connecticut, did a national survey that showed that only three percent of Americans had written specific long-range goals.[12] "They may have long-range goals swimming around in their heads, but nothing's going to happen until they jerk those nebulous goals out of the air, plant them in the wet cement out there, come back to today, do their homework, and start controlling the only increment of time over which they have any control: Right now....An unwritten goal is merely a wish."[13]

If you write out a goal, your brain thinks it, your hand writes it, your eyes see it, and, then, your subconscious and the universe begin to plan ways to make it happen. If you keep your goals where you can see them each day, you can determine if you are truly spending your time trying to accomplish them or if you value other things more. If the latter is true, change your goals and be honest with yourself. "Once we can decide on what is really important and pay the price for it in time and effort, we can accomplish great things."[14]

Put these goals where you can see them. Spend some time thinking about them each day, but don't become obsessed with or overly worried about them. Just do one little thing each day that moves you toward your goal. Once, I wrote down some things I wanted and forgot about the list. I came across the list several years later and was amazed and pleased to find that I was doing three out of the five items. "It was Pasteur who said, 'Chance favors the prepared mind.' The more you have been trying to decide what to do about your work, the more likely you are to find a solution when you least expect it."[15]

"The greatest difficulties in getting what we want in life are, first, figuring out what we really want, and, second, taking the first step. By writing down your dreams and goals, you can learn what you want, and in what order of importance."[16]

We have to live in the paradox of wanting and delaying gratification. However, as Richard Bolles writes in *What Color is Your Parachute?* "You have got to know what it is you want, or someone is going to sell you a bill of goods somewhere along the line that can do irreparable damage to your self-esteem, your sense of worth, and your stewardship of the talents God gave you."[17] Want what you want, and then expect to work to get it—not that it will just be handed to you. Give yourself permission to make the list. Then pull back and be happy with what you have while working toward what you want. If you can stand the tension, you'll get more of what you want than those who never stretch themselves to think about it. Without goals, you stagnate or go backwards. With goals, you are drawn toward exciting possibilities. If you run out of things to strive for, you lose your zest for living.

References

1. Bolles, R. *The Three Boxes of Life*. Berkeley, Calif.: Ten Speed Press, 1981, p. 354.

2. Leider, R. *Life Skills: Taking Charge of Your Personal and Professional Growth*. San Diego, Calif.: Pfeiffer & Company, 1994, p. 121.

3. Kaiser, L., Kaiser and Associates, Brighton, Colo., personal communication, 1996.

4. Leider, R., *op cit.*, p. 23.

5. Howard, W., and Howard, A. *Exploring the Road Less Traveled.* New York, N.Y.: Simon and Schuster, Inc., 1985, p. 10.

6. Progoff, I. *At a Journal Workshop.* New York, N.Y.: Dialogue House Library, 1975, p. 102.

7. *Ibid.*, p. 129.

8. Figler, H. *The Complete Job-Search Handbook.* New York, N.Y.: Henry Holt and Co., 1979, p. 231.

9. Sher, B., with Smith, B. *I Could Do Anything If I Only Knew What It Was.* New York, N.Y.: Bantam Doubleday Dell Publishing Group, Inc., 1994, p. 26.

10. Marion, P. *Crisis Proof Your Career.* New York, N.Y.: Berkeley Books, 1994, p. 49.

11. Maister, D. *Managing the Professional Service Firm.* New York, N.Y.: The Free Press, 1993, pp. 3-4.

12. Smith, H. *The 10 Natural Laws of Successful Time and Life Management.* New York, N.Y.: Warner Books, A Time Warner Company, 1994, p. 79.

13. *Ibid.*, pp. 82-83.

14. *Ibid.*, p. 105.

15. Figler, H., *op cit.*, p. 262.

16. Leider, R., *op. cit.*, p. 141.

17. Bolles, R. *The 1985 What Color is Your Parachute?* Berkeley, Calif.: Ten Speed Press, 1985, p. 82

Other Reading

Elbow, P. *Writing Without Teachers*. New York, N.Y.: Oxford University Press, Inc., 1973.

Work Sheets

Life Stepping Stones

My personal life stepping stones:

____

____

____

____

____

____

What was good about your stepping stones?

____

____

____

____

____

____

____

What was bad?

____

____

____

____

____

____

____

What do you wish you had done?

What do you wish you had not done?

Do you see some meaning or a pattern that makes sense to you?

Do you see a natural progression?

Future Planning

Planning your future: What do you want from life?

1. ____________________
2. ____________________
3. ____________________
4. ____________________
5. ____________________

First Want

What do you want?

What will you have to pay (sacrifice) to get it?

What might get in the way, be an obstacle to getting what you want?

Can you picture yourself already having it?

What one thing could you do today that would move you toward your goal?

What don't you want to do anymore?

What are your "Evil Secrets?"

Second Want

What do you want?

What will you have to pay (sacrifice) to get it?

What might get in the way, be an obstacle to getting what you want?

Can you picture yourself already having it?

What one thing could you do today that would move you toward your goal?

What don't you want to do anymore?

What are your "Evil Secrets?"

Third Want

What do you want? What will you have to pay (sacrifice) to get it?

What might get in the way, be an obstacle to getting what you want?

Can you picture yourself already having it?

What one thing could you do today that would move you toward your goal?

What don't you want to do anymore?

What are your "Evil Secrets?"

Fourth Want

What do you want?

What will you have to pay (sacrifice) to get it?

What might get in the way, be an obstacle to getting what you want?

Can you picture yourself already having it?

What one thing could you do today that would move you toward your goal?

What don't you want to do anymore?

What are your "Evil Secrets?"

Fifth Want

What do you want?

What will you have to pay (sacrifice) to get it?

What might get in the way, be an obstacle to getting what you want?

Can you picture yourself already having it?

What one thing could you do today that would move you toward your goal?

What don't you want to do anymore?

What are your "Evil Secrets?"

Chapter Four

Planning for Change

When you finish life-work planning, you may decide to make some career changes. Sayings abound about people's resistance to change: "The only people who welcome change are wet babies." "Every change is perceived as a loss by someone." "You can't change others; you can only change yourself." These words of wisdom remind us that change is not easy. What we may dislike most is the sense of being out of control.

Some changes can be planned for. You can plan to change your career, move to another city, send your children to college, or buy a house. Other changes just come up and grab us, and then we learn to cope. You figure out how to survive the change of losing a loved one or being fired from a job. "Even moving from one management position to another level within the same company is a significant change and will carry with it all of the need for transitional adaptation, common to major personal crises."[1] One of the great challenges of life is not to let the vulnerability we feel when change surprises us keep us from seizing the power we have and planning for the future as much as we can.

We need to regain a sense of power and control in turbulent times and plan for the future. I don't mean control in the sense of bossing people around or arrogantly lauding our position over others to make them feel small. I'm talking about controlling our own destiny as much as we can. We need to use our personal power, not overuse or abuse our positional power, and not fret about power we do not have.

You can gain some sense of control over change by planning ahead and visualizing how the change will affect you. The more you can picture what you'd like to do the more you can make it possible.

"As you begin to negotiate change in your life, keep in mind that you're entitled to disorganization and confusion. They are signs of health. Sometimes they are the side-effects that make you resistant to a change, even though you earnestly want the final outcome." Be patient with yourself and know the confusion will eventually subside and you will see the path clearer. "Changing can be a way of taking charge, of getting in the driver's seat, and of predicting your life's path while everything around you is unpredictable."[2]

In this chapter I'll discuss issues to think about if you are planning a career change and ways to continue what you are doing now but change your environment so you will be more satisfied.

Change Your Career

Before you make a career change, do some planning to make the transition go smoother. Think about the following issues:

Geography/Location

Where do you want to live? Is sunshine important to you or snow for cross country skiing? Do you like the wide open spaces of country living, or do you like to get to the grocery store or hardware store in five minutes? If the sight of miles and miles of cornfields gives you a feeling that all is right with the world, New York City will not be the place for you.

I like the tall trees, the rolling hills, and the brick houses where I grew up. I think we may be like baby ducks who choose as their mama the first animal they see. Our psyches tend to want to live in or get back to the kind of land we grew up in, if we had pleasant experiences there. Consider not fighting this urge—work on getting a job in the location you like best.

A couple from Arizona was interviewing for a job in the Northeast. The job, the schools, the house, the community all seemed right, but after two visits, something wasn't right, and they just couldn't figure it out. When they got back home, they realized the sun had not shone any time during their visits. They were used to seeing the sun every day, and they decided not to take the job. Sunshine was that important to them.[3]

Don't start with the notion that you will go anywhere in the country. You probably wouldn't be happy everywhere, and the thought is too broad to work with. Just as a history teacher told you to narrow your topic when you chose Russia as the subject for a term paper, pick a part of the country you like and then work to find a job there. If later, after a visit somewhere else, you decide the new place is all right, that's fine, but it's mind-boggling to start with the entire United States or the world in mind.

Health Issues

I have talked to people who have had a variety of health concerns. One person's arthritis improved in Arizona, but the dry weather there also caused another to suffer nosebleeds. One had circulation problems that worsened in extreme cold. Another's allergic reactions were continuous in the tropical warmth of Florida where something always blooms. Think about yourself and your family members. Will you be comfortable enough in the new location?

Life-Style

Life-style issues to consider are:

- Pace of life—Do you want to work from 8 a.m. to 6 p.m., or do you want to work from 6 a.m. to 9 p.m.? Many will say they do not have a choice. You always have choices. If two people drive a delivery truck and one works the night shift and the other the day shift, their life-styles are very different. Emergency department doctors and pediatricians have very different life-styles.
- Recreational opportunities—Do you want to play golf, sky dive, scuba dive, water or snow ski?
- Cultural events—Do you like opera, theater, ballet, foreign films?
- Social events—Do you want to belong to a country club, or do you prefer simple evenings at home with pizza and beer?
- Friends—In some areas, neighbors bring ice tea when you are unloading the moving van. In other areas, you can live there for years and never know your neighbor's name.

Financial Needs

I once talked to a physician who made about six to ten thousand dollars a year. In addition, he received room and board where he worked. He said, "If I make much more than that, I give it away. He travels between Alaska, the Pacific northwest, and Brazil throughout the year, giving his services away some of the time, making a modest salary other times. Variety, travel, and service to humanity are his most important values.

I talked to another physician who makes more than $200,000 and cannot get by on less. I am not asking you to pass judgment on yourself, but I am asking you to think hard about what amount you want and need and then make plans for how to get it.

Here are some questions to ask yourself:

- **What does it cost to live each month?** Make a list of the items.

  House payment
  Car payment
  Food
  Utilities
  Insurance
  Recreation
  Savings for college
  Clothing
  Vacation
  Taking care of parent

- **What could you change?** Baber suggests that you then "categorize your monthly expenditures:

  Fixed: rent, mortgage, car payments, utilities

  Flexible: food, clothing, education

  Frills: entertainment, club memberships, vacations[4]

  You probably can't change your house payment but could change clothes buying and recreation. A discussion of finances is often painful, because it kicks up a power struggle between partners—who decides how the money is spent. Is it shared equally? Should it be? Even though it is tough, make yourself talk about it. A fee-only financial planner, one who is selling nothing except advice, can be a big help, because he or she can help keep the conversation objective and give you advice without trying to sell you a product.

- **What amount of money do you have in a retirement fund?** What will it be worth when you retire? The time to begin planning your retirement finances is when you're young, when you have the years to build the "nest egg" you decide you'll need. If you desire an annual retirement income of $50,000, for instance, you'll need a fund of $715,000 to provide it without tapping the principal, presuming an interest rate of 7 percent.

  Some physicians want to keep working rather than retire, but I've talked to a number of physicians in their 60s who are having difficulty getting the jobs they want. Can you reduce your expenses when you retire? It would help if your house is paid for. "If you make even one extra mortgage payment a year, you can virtually cut a thirty-year mortgage in half—again, with big savings on interest."[5]

- **What do you make now?**

- **What will you make if you change jobs?** If you are going to step down in salary, can you try living on less for a couple of years to experience what it feels like and to build a financial cushion.

- **What severance benefits do you have and for how long?** Some people get as much as a full year of salary and benefits. Six months is nice. Three months is too little.

- **What new expenses can you anticipate for a job search?**

  "You will have new expenses during your job hunt: resume preparation, mailing, telephone, career counseling, health insurance, and memberships in professional associations if they previously were paid for by your employer."[6]

Experience

Organizations want medical directors who have experience. It's the age-old question of how do you get experience when everyone wants someone who already has experience. Volunteer to serve on and lead committees on utilization review, quality assurance, strategic planning, privileging, or credentialing. Sometimes HMOs and insurance companies will hire physicians part time to do utilization review and quality assurance. See if that opportunity is available in your area.

Find someone who is doing what you want to do and talk to them about it. What experience led them to where they are? To get the job you want, you may have to take a less than ideal job to get some marketable experience. Chapter 5 is devoted to how to get experience.

Educational Needs

Think about what education you will need to do the job you want. You can learn management skills through courses from ACPE, other organizations, or master's degree programs. Which ones suit your time schedules, finances, study habits?

If you decide to get a master's degree, keep in mind that it will definitely help you do a management job, but it will not be an automatic guarantee that you will get a management job. When you finished your MD, you could go somewhere and immediately be a doctor. The same is not true for the master's degree programs. You will still need experience and contacts.

Culture Shock

"Once they move into management, physician executives find that their former associates in practice consider them 'traitors' who have left a 'real job' and abandoned membership in a select professional clique....They may find their social network of physician friends no longer interested in their company and aloof to them."[7]

Physicians have told me that when they move into management, they are neither fish nor fowl. Their physician colleagues think they are now one of the administrators, and the administrators think they are still one of the physicians. They cope with this isolation by getting together with other physician executives. Several have formed organizations at the state or the local level. Many come to ACPE meetings primarily to be with like-minded people, and some keep in touch with other physician executives through regular phone calls.

Family Concerns

"Before signing on for a specific job, the physician should strongly consider the impact of this particular decision on the spouse and family. This includes issues such as relocation, a change in salary, uncertainty about the future, all of which could put great strain on family relationships. A physician executive is more likely to fail without good support from the 'home front.'"[8]

My husband was a practicing pediatrician who became more and more interested in medical management. He actively interviewed for positions for two years. Each time he went off to interview, I felt sick, because I did not want to leave Charlotte, North Carolina. I loved the town, my friends, the church, the schools; however, I knew I wouldn't be able to look at him years later and realize I kept him from doing something he had been working toward for so long. The city we lived in had only one large group and someone else had gotten that physician executive job. He interviewed in several places in the north and the midwest for two years before an offer came from Florida. Having been reared in the South I preferred going to warmer weather rather than colder weather. I finally agreed to go.

Then I was miserable and resentful for a year. My husband was excited about the new job and the new set of friends at work. The children and I cried a lot, but after two months the children had adjusted. I became lonelier and angrier. I had given up a good job in Charlotte and was having trouble filling my days with meaningful activity. After a year had passed, we talked to a counselor to help us tell each other what we needed. If this happens to your family, go sooner. We finally got there, but my suffering might have been shortened had we gone sooner. You need a third party to help you tell each other what you want and how you hurt. The counselor can help make suggestions for what might make you feel better. It's hard to think of these things on your own when you are in the middle of much pain and frustration.

The second year in Florida, I began going to graduate school to work on a PhD. I've always loved going to school. The university was a 100 miles away so I spent the night and took all the classes I could get in that 24-hour period. I enjoyed getting away from home, child care, and cooking once a week, and I felt some sacrifices were being made on my behalf—that cures resentment.

You need to communicate with your family. Are they willing to move with you and perhaps more than once? There are no guarantees, but you have a better chance if everyone is talking about it. Explain how excited you are about management, about making a difference on a larger scale rather than in one-on-one patient care, about being a part of the solutions to health care reform. Or you may explain that the need for your specialty is drying up, and you are going to be without income. Listen long and hard to objections, whining, crying, complaining. That is part of the price of uprooting your family. Say you're sorry they're in pain. Offer to be with the children on Saturday or help with the baby sitting so your spouse can do something he or she wants to do. I know you are busy and keeping long hours, but you must find time and something of yourself to give—not just money—if you want more cooperation and less resentment.

Whether married or single, carefully consider what your obligations are. Whom do you need to take care of? Whom do you want to live close to?

Should You Resign?

I have met a fair number of physicians who want to leave their situations as fast as they can. Marion has a tough list of questions to ask yourself before you quickly leave what you are doing now:

- "Do you have enough money to live for six months while you look?
- "Are all the other areas in your life fairly stable: your marriage, your finances, your debt-to-savings ratio, your relationship with your children, your feelings about yourself?
- "Are your moods consistent?
- "Do you feel capable of structuring your day when there is little or no external structure?
- "Do you like working out of your house alone most of the day?
- "Do you feel okay knowing that this is a three-to-six-month effort requiring six to eight hours a day?
- "Do you have supportive friends to help you through this process?
- "Do you have a network of 125 or more colleagues, friends, and co-workers or have what it takes to build one?
- "Do you have some good answers as to why you resigned?
- "Do you feel confident enough to handle the barrage of questions from recruiters, employers, and colleagues?

"If you can answer yes to most or all of these questions, it may be that you have sufficient structure in your life to go on your own. In this case, you may want to resign and work full time on your crisis-proof career."[9]

Change Your Environment

If you decide you can't leave your situation, changing your environment may help. You may decide you do not want to make a dramatic career change, but you want to make changes in your life so you are more satisfied. You do have choices in life. Even if you continue to do exactly what you are doing professionally, you have the choice of changing your attitude about it, of adding pleasurable experiences to your life, of reducing your work load so you have time for recreation. You need to ask yourself, "What plans can I (or have I) formulated to reduce...stress (e.g., exercise program, more sleep, more time off)?"[10] If you died tomorrow, life would go on somehow, so you might as well take some time off. If it means less money, what expenses could you cut back on to make that possible?

Pick one or two of the following to try. Schedule more free time or take up a new hobby. Take art, dance, or music classes. Help the homeless. Watch the Comedy Channel. Join a group that believes in a cause. Get a pet who will be affectionate and accept you as you are all the time.

Make time for exercise. You've heard that over and over again. If you are still not doing it, keep trying to make it happen. You simply cannot have a sense of well-being without exercise. The body was made to move, and if it doesn't get to, your mind, body, and spirit will suffer. Exercise can make you have or regain a sense of power. Slamming a golf ball far down the fairway can restore your feeling of control over some things. Running or walking fast gives you energy, releases frustration, and makes your body feel strong and slim.

Talk to Someone

Talk it over with someone, preferably a counselor. "You should seek professional intervention (such as psychotherapy) any time you become entrenched in a personal issue that is so intense or of such long duration that it affects your career....You don't have to be on the verge of a nervous breakdown to ask for help. A few short sessions may help you get unwedged."[11]

Family members eventually get worn out with the topic of your frustrations about health care changes and about career changes that you are considering. Also, they may feel frightened by these losses, so you may hold back some of your discontent. "The most resistance to switching jobs (or careers) often comes from colleagues or members of one's family who may feel threatened by a proposed change."[12]

A physician told me he would be ruined if he talked to a counselor. His insurance company would not cover him anymore if it learned he had had mental health counseling. If you worry about such repercussions, try a minister or a wise friend. Another option is to pay for these services yourself and not charge them to your insurance carrier. Some big group practices have private employee assistance programs just for their physicians. The CEO, who might insist that the physicians use the service, does not know what happens when they do. In many cases, the situations are improved and the process is completely confidential, and that is the CEO's only concern.

Separate whether you dread most how the change will affect you or how others will react to it. Will your spouse and children make you miserable because you are bringing in less money? How can you talk about it? Is there anything that can be done? Can you cut back on expenses? You might say to your family, ____ is happening. We have to cut back somewhere." Does everyone give up something or do you determine who gives up what? Often, it can't be a democratic family vote. Perhaps you decide a daughter must give up riding lessons or a son golf lessons. A teenager might get an afternoon job to finance some of the extras.

Find a support group—like-minded people who want to do an activity that you want to do or who want to complain about and problem solve issues that matter to you. Do you have people you can talk to about your life? For some, one on one is desirable. Others need a group to be with. Carl Jung, a late 19th and early 20th Century psychiatrist and philosopher, said that, for the well-balanced life, we need to tend to the inner and the outer life, but neither to the exclusion of the other. We can examine our inner selves when we are working or thinking alone, but we need a group or a community as a context for tending to the outer life. We need to interact with others, come up against their needs and wants, and use the energy of many ideas to get things done. Working with others in some way helps our own lives be centered, productive, healthy.

Write about It

You can tend to the inner life by writing in a journal for 10 minutes a day. You can write out some of these anxieties. Choose paper and pen you like or a computer and write 10 minutes a day, five days a week without worrying about spelling, grammar, or punctuation. Just start writing and don't stop for 10 minutes, whether you think you have anything to write about or not.

Write about the injustice of all the changes in health care. Lambaste the legal profession, the new managed care structures, ungrateful patients, whoever is causing longer hours and less money. When you do this kind of writing, you may touch on subjects that surprise you and that you wouldn't ever want anyone to see. If that happens, tear up the paper it is written on. You don't have to keep it to have the process benefit you. As Peter Elbow says, "Garbage in your head will poison you, but garbage on paper can safely be put in the wastepaper basket."[13] A physician recently took this suggestion and called to tell me he does the writing at the end of the day, and he has started sleeping better at night.

References

1. Hartfield, J. "Career Paths." In *Physicians in Managed Care. A Career Guide.* Bloomberg, M., and Mohlie, S., Editors. Tampa, Fla.: American College of Physician Executives, 1994, p. 72.
2. Wonder, J., and Donovan, P. *The Flexibility Factor.* New York, N.Y.: Ballantine Books, 1989, p. 6-7.
3. Bonfield, W. "It Took a Distant Opportunity to Show Us We Like It Where We Are." *Physician Executive* 14(5):8-11, Sept.-Oct. 1988
4. Baber, A., and Waymon, L. *How to Fireproof Your Career. Survival Strategies for Volatile Times.* New York, N.Y.: Berkley Books, 1995, p. 125.
5. *Ibid.*, p. 139.
6. *Ibid.*, p. 125.
7. Peters, R. *When Physicians Fail As Managers.* Tampa, Fla.: American College of Physician Executives, 1994, p. 14.

8. *Ibid.*, p. 38.

9. Marion, P. *Crisis Proof Your Career.* New York, N.Y.: Berkley Books, 1994, pp. 164-5.

10. *Ibid.*, p. 133.

11. *Ibid.*, p. 57.

12. Leider, R. *Life Skills*. San Diego, Calif.: Pfeiffer and Company, 1994, p. 83.

13. Elbow, P. *Writing Without Teachers*. London, England: Oxford University Press, 1973, p. 8..

Other Reading

Alexander, J. *Dare to Change*. New York, N.Y.: New American Library, 1984.

Covey, S. *The 7 Habits of Highly Effective People*. New York, N.Y.: Simon and Schuster, 1989.

Frankl, V. *Man's Search for Meaning*. New York, N.Y.: Washington Square Press, 1985. (First published in 1946.)

Gillett, R. *Change Your Mind. Change Your World*. New York, N.Y.: Simon and Schuster, 1992.

Seagrave, A., and Covington, F. *Free from Fears*. New York, N.Y.: Poseidon Press, 1987.

Wallen, E. "Job Pressures Seen Fueling Rise in Doctors' Stress Levels." *Physicians Financial News*, Oct. 15, 1993, pp. 15-16

Wheelis, A. *How People Change*. New York, N.Y.: Harper-Colophon Books, 1973.

Work Sheets

Personal Parameters of a Career Change

Geography/Location (list all of the conditions that you would impose on a move from your present location):

Health Issues (list considerations for all members of your family):

Life-Style (include, but do not limit yourself to, pace of life, recreational opportunities, cultural events, social events, and friends):

Financial Needs

Monthly Costs:

House payment ______________________________

Car payment ______________________________

Food ______________________________

Utilities ______________________________

Insurance ______________________________

Recreation ______________________________

Savings for college ______________________________

Clothing ______________________________

Vacation ______________________________

Taking care of parents ______________________________

Other ______________________________

Other ______________________________

Other ______________________________

Other ______________________________

Other ______________________________

Total ______________________________

What would you change? (categorize your monthly expenses)

Fixed ______________________________

____

____

____

Flexible ______________________________

____

____

____

Retirement funds (list current funds and projected funds for anticipated retirement years. In constructing a financial retirement package, remember that you will want to live on the interest on your retirement fund principal. For instance, the annual income at 7 percent interest on a fund of $715,000 is $50,000. If you will require more income, the principal must be increased by $143,000 for each income increase of $10,000.):

Current funds ____________________

Funds ___ years from now ____________________

Funds ___ years from now ____________________

Funds ___ years from now ____________________

Funds ___ years from now ____________________

Funds ___ years from now ____________________

Anticipated salary in new job ____________________

Severance and other benefits (amount and term)

____________________ ____________________

____________________ ____________________

____________________ ____________________

____________________ ____________________

____________________ ____________________

____________________ ____________________

Job Search Expenses

Resume preparation____________________

Mailing and shipping____________________

Telephone ____________________

Career counseling ____________________

Health insurance ____________________

Membership dues____________________

Other____________________

Other____________________

Other____________________

Other____________________

Checklist for Resignation (if you respond positively (Y) to most of these questions, you can probably sustain yourself and your family for the six months or so needed to find another position. Otherwise (N), hunt from where you are)

- Do you have enough money to live for six months while you look?_____
- Are all the other areas in your life fairly stable: your marriage, your finances, your debt-to-savings ratio, your relationship with your children, your feelings about yourself? _____
- Are your moods consistent?_____
- Do you feel capable of structuring your day when there is little or no external structure?_____
- Do you like working out of your house alone most of the day?_____
- Do you feel okay knowing that this is a three-to-six-month effort requiring six to eight hours a day?_____
- Do you have supportive friends to help you through this process?_____
- Do you have a network of 125 or more colleagues, friends, and co-workers or have what it takes to build one?_____
- Do you have some good answers as to why you resigned?_____
- Do you feel confident enough to handle the barrage of questions from recruiters, employers, and colleagues?_____

Chapter Five

What Do You Have to Do to Become a Physician Executive?

Physicians who are considering moving from clinical practice into management often ask, "What do you have to do to make the change?"

◆ **Become a board-certified clinician who practices three-five years.**

Residents who are interested in management and who do not want to practice clinically have asked, "Why do I need to be board certified when I am not going to practice?" As a medical director you will be working with physicians, in some cases telling them what they can and cannot do. Physicians respect other physicians most for their knowledge of disease and their capacity to take care of patients. Only gradually do they come to respect them for their management skills. They will not take instructions from someone who has not had to cope with an overcrowded schedule, shrinking resources, government regulations, the threat of malpractice suits, and night call, to name a few of the frustrating realities of being a practicing clinician.

You do not have to practice full time, but it has to be a setting where you are fully responsible for some patients. Nancy Ashbach, MD, MBA, says, "The clinical experience is critical—five years of it but not necessarily full time. Urgent care facilities where you haven't had full responsibility for patients are not as good as half time for Kaiser or half time for a group," she says.[1]

◆ **Get management experience.**

Serve on committees and task forces. Let people see you doing management activities, working with people and tackling problems. If you serve on and/or lead the long-range planning committee, the utilization review and quality assurance committee, the credentialing committee, you can claim all of them as experience when you are ready to move more into management.

Get involved in the county medical society, the state medical society, the American Medical Association. Some HMOs and insurance companies hire people to do utilization review and quality assurance part time. This is valuable experience for a management career.

"If you think you might be interested in hospital management, you would be wise to do what you can to move up in the elected or selected hierarchy of your hospital medical staff. Express interest in becoming chair of your clinical department or be willing to serve on the hospital executive committee. Be available to take a job as an elected officer of the hospital staff. The same would be true for those aspiring to positions in management in medical group practices or various types of HMOs."[2]

I know a Florida physician who has been part of a team that is planning a state HMO. He said that, if you had asked him six months ago if he would be involved in such a project, he would have said no. Some physicians are helping with the formation of the many physician-hospital organizations that are jockeying to get in place. You might volunteer to work with your hospital, group practice, or IPA on outcomes monitoring projects.

Many men and women go into management in the middle of their careers. They may reach the point where they feel they have done all the cardiovascular surgery they want to do, or they can't discuss otitis media one more time. It is no longer a challenge, and they need a new challenge. Because many people come to the point in their careers that they want a change, volunteer for committees throughout your career to continually learn new activities, to make yourself visible in the organization, and to have experience to put on your résumé should you decide management appeals to you some day.

You may have to take a management job that is not quite right in order to get the necessary experience. Once you go into the management arena, you may have to move every three to five years. You need to think about whether you want to do that.

- **Get education.**

The Physician in Management seminars of the American College of Physician Executives are an excellent source of training in basic management skills. Attend the College's Institutes, which have even more concentrated areas of study. Be on the alert for informal educational opportunities from other national professional organizations and from local colleges and universities. Get a master's degree if you have the time and financial resources.

- **Find a mentor.**

Roger Schenke, ACPE Executive Vice President, advises: "Find yourself a mentor—male or female. Someone who has experience, who will help you think. Look for someone who is an effective person. If you admire the person and think you would like to be more like him or her, try to get on a committee that the person is on, or in an educational program that the person is in. Get in the same room, get to know the person. It will be natural for the conversation to be around management issues. Then ask: 'How does someone get involved in management in this organization? How did you get to where you are? Has this management change been good for you? What education did you get?' If that person sees you begin to do management activities, he or she becomes like your mother or father because he or she helped to get you started."[3]

Mentoring takes less time than many people think. The person does not have to be in your organization or even in your town. You can call them and say, "Can you listen to me for a while? 20-30 minutes."

Mentoring does not have to be regular. I have heard people try to set up formal situations—a contract where I'll help you with your weakness and you help me with mine. Once in a while that might work, but a formal commitment to a specific amount of time can scare people off. They may give you that much time because they get interested in you, but they don't want to promise it.

In some companies, mentor situations exist where someone spends a considerable amount of time at another company—at another hospital in the same hospital system or at another staff model in the same managed care system. A new medical director can be sent to the site and walk around with an experienced medical director for a week and learn how he or she does things.

"Information interviews are valuable and may be the beginning of a mentoring relationship. There are two types. First, you can have an information interview with a physician in management who has a job that you think you would like. For instance, if you are interested in group practice management, interview several physicians who are medical directors in group practices. These information systems may lead to a long-term mentor relationship."[2]

"A second type of information interview would be one in which you interview someone who works for an organization that you might like to work for. If you desire an information interview with a health care executive in a large insurance company, plan two or three questions that you would ask that person and tell them ahead of time that you do not intend to take more than 15 minutes of their time. You should have the key questions written out so you could at least get them answered if there is not time to get other questions dealt with. Of course, if you already know the person, it would be all right to expect a longer interview or possibly an interview over lunch that you pay for."[2]

Don't continue a mentoring relationship if sexual stuff gets in the way. It is very natural for people who work together to become good friends. The sparks of creativity generated by good minds thinking together can sometimes lead to sexual thoughts. If either person acts on these thoughts, it is wise to end a mentoring relationship. The trouble you can get into can outweigh any benefits you might receive.

Kaiser says, "[W]e are all mentors for the people who have not moved as far on the path as we have, and at the same time we are dependent on mentors who are further along on the journey to help us take the next step....You may never be able to help the people who help you. Your service is to those who are coming along behind you."[4]

How Some Physician Executives Gained Experience

Peters describes the dual nature of the physician executive's role. "The job dimensions of physician managers...are of a 'clinical' nature—evaluating physician performance, utilization and case review, recruiting physicians and defining their clinical activities, and quality of care considerations. Other tasks are of a more 'managerial' nature—planning, budgeting, marketing, and cost of care considerations."[5] You will need experience in both areas before you can get a full-time position.

At a focus group I conducted in 1996 at a meeting of the American College of Physician Executives, I asked five physicians how they had gotten management experience. The following summaries highlight their answers.

John O'Malley, MD, FACPE, Senior Vice President, System Clinical Services, Louisiana Health Services Corporation, Lafayette

The first management position I had was director of consultation at the Children's Hospital in Boston. I was to put the services together and meet the needs of the general hospital. That gave me some introduction to coordinating people and schedules, talking people into doing things. My second position was medical director of a new adolescent psychiatric hospital. It involved more people, more tasks, a lot of support from hospital administrators. Then I became vice president of a national mental health company. I talked to people who had gone through the same process before.

Since January 1996, I've been Senior Vice President for Louisiana Health Systems, a conglomeration of acute care hospitals, nursing homes, urgent care centers, and other facilities. I obtained my current position on the basis of experience. The number of years that I spent in Philadelphia in those multiple tasks involved many skills that have been picked up one by one. I did not seek an advanced degree until now. I am in a master of health administration program at the University of Colorado.

Knowledge of how to provide staffing coverage for a variety of hospitals and physicians came from other physicians and administrators who had done it for a long time. I watched them sit down and put a schedule together, prepare a budget. A finance course does not help you do a budget. What helps me do a budget is other people who have done it for 19 years showing me how to do it or pointing out that I haven't allocated money for such and such. It was a mentorship from a variety of people who already had those skills—both physicians and administrators—people who have been in the business for a long time.

John R. Sanders, MD, Vice President, Medical Staff Services, Greenville Hospital System, Greenville, South Carolina

Since January 1996, I've been Vice President of Medical Staff Services for a local hospital. I've been an orthopedist for 20 years in Greenville, South Carolina. For 20 years, I've been on every committee there is. Every time something came up, I either volunteered or got appointed to it. Sometimes I unvolunteered myself, but too many times I didn't know how to say no. I had mentoring from individuals who had put budgets and plans together. I gained skills about strategic planning, whether it be for programs, departments, blending departments, or fighting battles of cross-credentialing. You learn people skills and coping skills. It's the school of hard knocks. I've gone to a few courses here and there, but I've not had formal MBA training.

N. L. "Sax" Saxton, MD, FACPE, Vice President, Medical Affairs, Antelope Valley Hospital Medical Center, Lancaster, California

I've been a Vice President of Medical Affairs in California 1½ years. I've been a medical director for 17 years, and this is my fourth hospital. I went from private practice of 11 years into academic medicine in Texas. It was during that time that I began doing tasks that had minor administrative responsibilities—scheduling, working out conflict between residents and faculty.

The thing that helped me the most during that time was I became a leader in the Boy Scouts. It has a program called Woodbadge that is its highest level of adult training. It teaches adults how to teach young people. It teaches 11 competencies—counseling, setting an example, running meetings, etc., all during two weeks of training in outdoor survival. They are the same skills that are being taught in business management training programs. Without realizing it, I was in a management training course. I needed to learn more about those skills, so I started taking courses with the American College of Physician Executives. I've been coming to its meetings for 17 years.

Gary Fleming, MD, Director, Medical Affairs, Athens Regional Medical Center, Athens, Georgia

At the hospital where I practiced medicine, the newest guy in became chairman of the department, so I became chair of the Department of Pediatrics. It gave me an opportunity to be at executive committee meetings with the CEO of the hospital. The sister, who was CEO of the Catholic hospital, soon found out I was interested in how mentally handicapped people were taken care of in

Western Maryland at that time. She invited me to be on the Board of the Mental Health Advisory for the County Commissioners. She was influential in my being selected chairman after a couple of years. She was a mentor. When we established a mental health facility in Allegheny County, Maryland, she stressed two things. One was KISS—Keep it simple, stupid. To exemplify, when we were making our presentations to the governor and the state legislature, we made it as simple as possible. She also emphasized the sheepdog form of leadership, where, if you expect the medical staff to do anything, you have to talk one-on-one to them. When they are all moving in the right direction, you move around in front of them. The technique acknowledges the truism that a leader cannot lead without followers. It was the mentoring of this administrator that taught me management skills and helped me get the necessary experience to become a medical director. She was pleasantly upset when I wound up being the medical director for a competing hospital in the same area.

Randy Ellis, MD, FACPE, Clinical Director, ProMed, Inc., Charlotte, North Carolina

I am Clinical Director for ProMed in Charlotte, North Carolina—ambulatory care units that do about 50 percent acute care and 50 percent occupational medicine.

I fell into my first management job sort of by default. You take a job and suddenly they give you administrative tasks to do because you are the only one who will do the paperwork. You are the one who is suddenly going to the committees and writing the policies and trying to do the quality assurance. I did a lot of work in utilization review, in cost containment.

I became medical director of an emergency department where we saw 57,000 patients a year, and I had a staff of 20 physicians. I had no management training. I worked for a company that staffed emergency departments. The hospital saw me as being nonadministration. The medical staff saw me as being administration. The company saw me as out there in Podunk, and nobody was interested in training me.

I said "I've got to learn something here," so I started going to Career Track seminars on presentations, communication skills, management styles. That's how I started picking up skills. Later, I heard about the American College of Physician Executives and began attending its classes. That's where I began a lot of my formal training in management.

Having presented the ways in which these five physician executives got their experience, I want to end this chapter with a wish list that an organization gave to a recruiter for the qualities it wanted in its next medical director. Organizations want physician executives to have experience handling the problems associated with the many changes in health care, but they also want strong communication skills, which will be discussed in the next chapter.

1. We need someone who will not say one thing and do another.

2. The medical director must help us understand where administration stands on various issues.

3. The person must demonstrate consistency and fairness.

4. The physician must have the ability to stand up to special selfish interests on the medical staff. (e.g., orthopedists who won't take trauma call even when the by-laws are clear on that issue.)

5. The medical director will help us with all the transitional stress, such as personnel needs, downsizing, consolidation of medical staffs.

6. The person will develop managed care agreements that protect all parties.

7. We still have lots of room for improvement in reducing lengths of stays.

8. The person must be strong on quality.

9. The medical director must have significant managed care experience, but that is not as important to us as the willingness to learn that stuff and teach it to us.

10. Some doctors feel that they are being told what to do by administration. If the medical director can break down some of that feeling, he or she will win a lot of points.

11. If the medical director can help us deal with some of our problem staff members, he or she will gain credibility right away.

12. More important to us than technical skills are personal traits—warm and friendly, a diplomat, a good communicator (by that we mean someone who is good at listening, explaining, and convincing).

References

1. Nancy Ashbach, MD, MBA, Network Medical Director, MetLife of Colorado, Denver, personal communication, 1992.

2. George E. Linney Jr., MD, FACPE, Vice President, Tyler & Company, Atlanta, Georgia, personal communication, 1992.

3. Roger Schenke, Executive Vice President, American College of Physician Executives, Tampa, Florida, personal communication, 1992.

4. Kaiser, L. *Lifework Planning*. Brighton, Colo.: Brighton Books, 1989, p. 7.

5. Peters, R. *When Physicians Fail As Managers*. Tampa, Fla.: American College of Physician Executives, 1994, p. 6.

Chapter Six

What Communication Skills Have You Needed Most in Your Job?

I asked experienced physician executives what communication skills have been most useful in their management positions. In this chapter you will read their responses and then a discussion of the most needed communication skills.

John O'Malley, MD, FACPE, Senior Vice President, System Clinical Services, Louisiana Health Services Corporation, Lafayette

Physicians, as a group, are not easily led in one direction or another. If I need to get something done that may be tinged with some controversy, I go to the leaders first, one on one, and work out whatever concerns they may have. I get their support and then go on to get the support of others. I've tried it other ways, but they haven't worked. It's salesmanship. It's understanding where they are coming from, what their concerns are. I listen through what their complaints are. Often their complaints are not the real issue.

Being able to address a group is very important—to give key ideas and get people fired up to know what needs to be done.

Writing skills are also important—everything from writing a memo to writing an article for the local newspaper to writing a newsletter about the future of medicine and American health economics.

John Sanders, MD, Vice President, Medical Staff Services, Greenville Hospital System, Greenville, South Carolina

You need to listen and listen and listen. When I was in training, the chief used to say, "If all else fails, try listening to patients. They are trying to tell you what's wrong." The same is true for the groups who are bringing you problems.

When my girls were teenagers, I took a parenting course called active listening. If you tell me the sky is blue, I might say, You think the blue color of the sky is pretty. It's a way of sending back a message that you are indeed hearing what the other person is saying and then they feel more comfortable. It worked with the kids. It often works with the "children" on the medical staff.

Don't be afraid to say you don't know. You probably know about a book on the subject or about someone who has been there before, so you can figure out where to get the information. Crucial is follow up. Just as with a patient who has a problem, get back with them and say, I found such and such. I'm not happy with what I've found so far, but we are still looking. Do you have any ideas? Have you talked to anyone else about this? Follow up is important.

Chalmers M. Nunn Jr., MD, Vice President of Medical Affairs, Nash General Hospital, Rocky Mount, North Carolina

I'm a salesman. I have to sell a new product to our physicians who don't want to buy it. When you are selling to doctors, it requires a lot of one-on-one and small group conversations, because they won't buy that product unless you really convince them. You need the qualities it takes to be a salesman—energy, excitement. For example, I work a lot with pathways, guidelines, and quality improvement. I had to convince the orthopedic surgeons to really get tough on their prosthetic salesmen and try to get the price down on their products. I said, "This is important to the hospital. I know it doesn't seem to affect you directly, but the more we can get their price down, the better off we are going to be in the long run and the better we will be able to be competitive down the road." When I showed them information about how their salaries were going down and the salesmen's salaries were going up to the point that, in less than 5 years, the salesmen were going to be making more than orthopedic surgeons, overnight these guys changed. You have to know what hits their buttons. I did that through reading the literature and finding confirmation of the point I was trying to put across.

The other thing I have to work hard at is anger control. I've always been pretty good at it, but I had to get better. Those of us in management have already made a major shift in thinking, but many physicians may not have changed their thinking. I have to catch myself so I don't speak too soon. When they are saying something that I know is totally wrong, I just have to bite my tongue. I have to exert that self-control and realize that now is not the time to speak. I don't have enough information, and what I say now will drive them in a direction I don't want them to go. I have to work very hard at that kind of calmness.

I work a lot at pulling teams together. Teams of people who have never worked with one another. Male physicians and a lot of female professionals. Most hospital roles are filled by women—nurses, physical therapists, respiratory therapists. It seems to me, when I'm having a meeting to develop a pathway, the group consists of two or three male doctors and ten female staff. You have to learn how to be an interpreter, a calmer of the meeting, how to keep the sexist language out of it that turns people off. I sometimes find that to be a significant problem, particularly with older members of the staff or with members of the staff from non-U.S. cultures.

What taught me the most about listening was being on the school board. I learned early on that the more I spoke the more trouble I got into. We had a meeting the other night, and it was obvious that one of the board members was politically attacking an employee. It had more to do with the who than the what and why, and I made the mistake of pointing that out in the meeting. In retrospect I thought I probably shouldn't have said anything. It didn't gain me anything, and probably raised the hackles even more. Two or three days later, I swallowed my pride a little and talked to this person again and rephrased the situation to defuse it. I think quite often we don't realize that we always have a second chance. We need to take advantage of it. We were taught in the College's power and influence course that we need to do what's uncomfortable in order to influence someone. In our communication, we have to do what is very uncomfortable to get the point across.

N.L. "Sax" Saxton, MD, FACPE, Vice President, Medical Affairs, Antelope Valley Hospital Medical Center, Lancaster, California

Listening is important, and it's hard for doctors to do that. We think people are asking our opinions, and we get carried away with giving it to them. Often, they want us to agree with them, and we haven't found out what their side of it is. When I'm listening and I want to talk, I try to listen for the things I can agree with. No matter how far apart we are, I try to find something I can agree with, so the first thing out of my mouth is something we agree on.

Writing is important. A lack of ability here can hurt you if you are talking about memos. In my first management position, I was pretty tickled with my title, and I liked sending out memos. I found I am easily misunderstood in writing. In speaking, I can almost sense when I've gone off on the wrong track, and I can readjust myself. Now most of the memos I write are signed by the chief of staff or the department chairs.

The ability to speak is also very important and there are all kinds of ways to improve those skills. When I first became a medical director, speaking in front of a group was a most frightening thing.

John O'Malley, MD, FACPE

Our entire management staff took a course on making presentations. During that first course, my hands shook and the papers rattled, but you gradually get over that. After 17 years, what makes my job easy is not having to go through such lengths to prepare, because almost everything I do I've done before.

Another communication skill that is necessary, especially as we bring groups together, is the ability to facilitate, to get the message from those who are quieter. I've learned from one-on-one conversations that some of those with the most to say, say the least in a group.

Gary Fleming, MD, Director, Medical Affairs, Athens Regional Medical Center, Athens, Georgia

An important communication skill is the ability to remain cool in body language. If someone is yelling obscenities at you, you need to try not to have body language that matches the person yelling at you.

As an example, I was confronted with a problem surgeon who knew all the answers. This surgeon had a big ego; he was very articulate, very well trained. The department chief demanded that we strip this surgeon of his clinical privileges, kick him off the medical staff because of his bad behavior. I was able to maintain my cool and encouraged the department chief to keep his cool when he confronted this surgeon. When the surgeon's behavior was articulated calmly and reasonably to the surgeon by the department chief, the surgeon voluntarily left our medical staff. Apparently, he was too enbarassed by his own behavior to remain active at our hospital. It is my understanding that his behavior at another hospital did subsequently improve (an attitude adjustment?).

Randy Ellis, MD, FACPE, Clinical Director, ProMed, Inc., Charlotte, North Carolina

Active listening and maintaining your cool are also very pertinent for a woman who wants to be a physician executive. A woman has to face different attitudes. Many times, male physicians will treat female physicians with the same cavalier attitude that they treat a nurse or receptionist or any other female who is working in a subservient role. Male physicians will come into a room and think that there are no physicians in the room if everyone is female. They will start the power game of yelling. Yelling works with women. You pound the table a little bit, and women will start to back off, because we are taught to not be confrontational. We are taught to be consensus builders and negotiators and often that is turned against us. We have to work through that in order not to back down and to face that confrontational situation. Being able to communicate your way through that behavior sometimes requires standing toe to toe with them. They have to learn that type of behavior is not going to make you back down. Often it only takes one or two episodes, and you never have to face that situation with that person again.

N.L. "Sax" Saxton, MD, FACPE

It's not just a gender thing. There is a female and a male style among physicians, regardless of gender. This distinction is very noticeable between surgeons and primary care physicians. Primary care physicians have more of a female style, more participative, more team-oriented.

The communication skills mentioned most often by these physician executives were: listening, talking one-on-one, using appropriate body language, making presentations, pulling teams together in meetings, dealing with conflict, and writing. In the next section, I'll suggest strategies for improving each of these skills.

Listening

Milo Frank says he asked a group of people how long they could pay attention to what someone was saying without letting their minds wander off to sex, money, or the other good things in life. He got "answers of anywhere from four hours to four seconds."[1] Listening takes enormous energy and discipline.

If you decide you are willing to expend the energy to listen, here are some techniques that will help you listen so people will want to give you important information and value you as a person who helps them solve problems:

- **Be quiet.** You cannot be listening if you are talking or if you are thinking hard about what you are going to say next. If you get very anxious about not knowing what to say when the person finishes, try putting all your energy into listening and then tell him or her, "I need to think about this. Can I get back with you in a while to talk more?"

  Roger Ailes, who coached President Bush during his presidential campaign, suggests that you should listen carefully before all interactions, particularly ones where you are scheduled to make a presentation. "When you enter a communication situation, don't immediately stand up and start projecting your voice and throwing out your opinions. Stop for a second, absorb what's going on. What's the mood of the room, the crowd—are they down, up, happy, expectant? Read what people are feeding back to you. Are they skeptical or eager?"[2] The only way to find this out is to be quiet and listen.

- **Use your body to let the person know you are there.** Look at him or her. Don't let your eyes wander all over the room. Sit attentively but not tensely, not slouching or lying down. On the sofa watching TV or reading the paper are not good positions for listening. Neither is opening your mail in your office while someone tries to tell you something. You may think you can do both, but the talker does not think you are listening and will be irritated.

- **Give an occasional "uh huh" or nod** to let the person know you are following his or her train of thought. If you are not, ask a question before you let the person go on too long and you are really lost.

- **Ask nonjudgmental questions.** "Can you say a little more? I'm not sure I understand. Will you try me again? What do you think that you'll do next?" Don't ask, "Why on earth did you do that?" There is absolutely no decent answer to that question, and the person doing the asking is implying, "You are an idiot!" You may be right, but if you want communication to continue, you will have to discipline yourself not to say everything you think.

Good listening requires asking timely questions that help the person along with the story. "Think of the people you know whom you consider to be true leaders. When you are with them, they invariably ask questions. They are interested in you and your ideas. They are also interested in improving their listening skills."[3]

- **Restate some of what the person has said** to demonstrate that you understand. For example, "You think the nurses on the floor resent the patient coordinators because they don't do shift work anymore?" This is not necessary in every situation. Sometimes questions that ask for more information let the person know you are with them.

- **Make a guess about a feeling** you think the person is having if it seems appropriate. "I can see why that would make you sad." They may reply, "I'm not sad, I'm angry." It doesn't matter if you are wrong. They will correct you, and you have gotten to a deeper level of communication when you find out how someone feels about a subject. They will feel a sense of relief and sometimes release when they identify the feeling.

  If someone describes an automobile accident to you, your reply of "That must have been frightening" lets them know you may have felt that too. Often, we feel alone when we have negative feelings, as if no one else has felt them. There is great comfort in knowing someone else has lived through them.

Listening becomes even tougher in heated emotional situations when people are angry. Sometimes people come to your office obviously upset. If you are feeling strong and collected, it is helpful if you can let the emotional person vent for a few moments. You might then respond, "I can see that you are angry, and I'm not surprised. What can I do to help?" If you are not up to being in the presence of so much negative energy, you might say, "I'll be glad to talk about this when you are calmer."

Don't do the following activities until you have spent a significant time listening:

- Don't give advice.

- Don't pass judgment.

- Don't tell your own experience.

As a physician executive, you are paid to give advice and pass judgment, but it's a matter of timing. We tend to want to do these three behaviors quickly. Save them for last, after you have let the person talk for a while.

Talking One on One

Robert Jamplis, MD, President and Chief Executive Officer of the Palo Alto Medical Foundation, Palo Alto, California, describes a time when he wanted to convince his group of physicians to do something that would cost them a lot of money, but would benefit the organization in the long term. "We individually went out and talked to every single partner. It took us six months, with dinners and everything else. We had 130 partners. We just pounded this in, and we finally got a unanimous vote."[4]

When you are in a one-on-one conversation:

◆ **Use the right amount of energy.**

Pronounce your words clearly. Also, do not use a voice that is too loud. Listeners will try to get away from you if you do. Don't mumble or slur your words. Use whatever energy it takes to get your words across to the other person. The listener should not have to struggle to hear you or understand you.

◆ **Avoid arrogance.**

"[A]rrogance combined with ego is a barrier to managerial effectiveness....[O]ne physician was quoted as saying: 'I am a doctor of medicine and obviously my field is more difficult and more important than management. I know that my field is more important because it requires years of study to become qualified; one can become a manager by simple organization appointment and without special education. Therefore, not just anyone can practice in my field but anyone can indeed practice management. Management is a lesser function than my own, so if I can successfully practice my own specialty, I must readily be able to manage—and manage better than most managers. I thus transfer my level of expertise to any field that is of lesser difficulty than my own specialty.' Thus, the conviction of some physicians that medicine is superior to management is often coupled with the assertion that it is easy to transfer one's medical expertise and experience to administration and human resources management. Of all the personal factors mentioned that hinder one's management career, this is perhaps the most 'deadly' flaw.'"[5]

Your word choice, your tone of voice, the position of your head and eyes can all convey arrogance. If you are thinking how much smarter and better you are than the person you are talking to, there is a good chance that message will come through, even if your words are satisfactory. If you find yourself thinking in this way, try changing to this thought, "What will it cost me if I alienate this person?"

◆ **Let the other person also talk.**

Don't talk longer than a couple of minutes without letting the other person talk. An important part of speaking effectively is not speaking too much. "If most of the time you talk more than you listen, you're probably failing in your communication and probably boring people, too."[6]

Taking turns was a valuable thing to learn in preschool, and we never outgrow the need to do it. I've had people say, "Why should I give you a turn, if you can't fight to say what you want to say." Remember that extroverts talk and then figure out what they think; introverts figure out what they think and then talk. Introverts have valuable information if you give them the air time to say it.

Extroverts sometimes talk too much. If you go on and on when you talk, people dread being around you. When they have to come to your office for a business conversation, they plan ways to get out before they ever come in. Jacquelyn Wonder, in *The Flexibility Factor*, described a cure for a client who talked too much in meetings. He drew on paper an imaginary tongue depressor divided into four parts. He could speak four times in a meeting and then no more. He had a hard time controlling himself at first, but he finally accomplished his goal. Eventually, he didn't need the image of the tongue depressor on paper but carried it in his mind. Six months later, he said, "This is one of the most valuable changes I've ever made. I've found that I get so much more out of a meeting by listening to others. I'd always felt responsible for rushing in and filling gaps in conversation and responding to a lecturer. Now I don't feel the tension I used to when there was a moment of silence. I'm more apt to see the big picture than before, and I recall the meeting as a whole, rather than just bits and pieces."[7]

I have also recommended to people that they squeeze one hand with the other to remind them of a change they want to make. The mild pain is a signal to the brain not to keep talking.

Suppose you don't speak up enough. Before you go into a meeting or a conversation, write out what you might say on a particular issue. You will not read it, but if you have focused your thoughts beforehand, you are more willing to risk your ideas. Then set a goal for yourself to speak at least twice during the session. Put a check on the notes in front of you each time you speak. If you have trouble speaking up on an unexpected topic that is being discussed, pretend to take notes about what others are saying, but really write down what you'd like to say. Once you see what you've written and see that it makes good sense, you will be more willing to say it to the group.

◆ **Be concise.**

Suppose you want to tell someone something he or she does not want to hear. You have a list of 18 things they have done wrong. Don't tell them all of them. Pick two or three.

Go in and say, "I am hearing complaints from the people in the accounting department. Do you want to hear about them?" Then tell two or three things—not 18. Prioritize them. You don't say, "Everyone is mad at you because you don't treat them with respect." Instead be specific and say, "When Jim came to talk to you about the budget, he said you interrupted him after two sentences and said, "You are crazy if you think I'm going to give you that much money."

Body Language

What causes someone to understand you and respond well to you? Research suggests that:

- 7 percent of understanding depends on the words you use.
- 38 percent depends on your tone of voice.
- 55 percent depends on your nonverbal body language.

"The reality is that few people accept responsibility for anything more than their words. They have never learned that a harsh tone can deny the gentlest of words."[8] Inappropriate body language can negate your message. "I'm not angry" said loudly while you're pounding on a table changes the meaning of the message.

Don't point constantly when you talk or make any strange gesture repeatedly. Look at yourself on videotape to see if you have any odd mannerisms or make any unpleasant sounds. It is amazing how unaware we can be. I've seen people scratch places repeatedly that should only be touched in private. I've heard people say "uhm" so much that I began to count them.

What constitutes a good voice and good body language?

- **Voice**

  "A positive voice is: cheerful, satisfied, concerned, warm," confident.

  "A negative voice is: sarcastic, scared, depressed, clipped, tense, too loud or soft.

- **Face and Body**

  "Positive face has: smile, occasional head nod, and eye contact.

  "Negative face has: frown, smirk, boring glare," wandering eyes.

  "Positive body language is: relaxed, leaning forward some, open arms.

  "Negative body language is: pointing, wandering eyes, picking at body."[9]

Tone of voice and body language are important when you have to fire someone. When someone has to be let go, you need to get out of the frame of mind that views it as a depressing, devastating event. You need to rise above the despair and say, in a calm, confident tone of voice, "You are a good person who has worked hard, but your strengths are not matching what we need to have done in this position. We failed to pick this up in the interview. Your strengths as a writer and editor are valuable and you need to find a place where those are called upon. We will help you in the future, give you good recommendations. We will give you this much severance."

Presentations

A recent survey found that some people fear public speaking more than death. But for those willing to do it, there is great satisfaction in having an audience respond well to a talk you've given. It also makes money for your organization. When people see a physician or a physician executive make an impressive speech in the community, they often will come to your group for medical care.

The first step in speech preparation is to think about the people who will be listening to you. When you make a talk, you are selling yourself to your audience. In order to sell anything, you have to find out what people want. To do that, you must analyze your audience: Are they male, female, young, old, a mixture? What's their cultural background? Will they understand your technical terms? If not, define them in a pleasant, noncondescending voice.

Pay attention to the language you use. Avoid unnecessary words and do not use overly long sentences. Generally, one idea per sentence is good. Figures of speech add color and excitement. ("Working in an emergency department is like walking through a mine field—one trauma exploding through the door after another." Or, "My life is like a roller coaster—up one minute and down the next.)

Unless you are very comfortable making speeches, write out exactly what you are going to say. Write it in a conversational style—not like an academic paper. Do not read the speech. Memorize it or learn it well enough that you do not say "um" while you are thinking of the next thing to say. Writing out the full speech reduces the "ums" of thinking time. When you know the speech well, your mind is freed of anxiety, and you will be able to add interesting examples to prove your points as you watch the reactions of the audience.

When you deliver the speech, stand erect with feet firmly on the floor. Don't lean on the flipchart stand or sit on a table. Look like you have the strength to be up there and entertain them. Use some gestures but not too many. Nothing is more distracting than watching someone who has just taken a course on public speaking and has added enough gestures to their talk to look like an ensign giving signals on a ship. Make direct eye contact with someone in each third of the room, slowly rotating your attention but in a random fashion. If you have the courage to look directly at a few people, the audience thinks you are confident.

Learn the beginning of the speech particularly well. That is when you are the most nervous and don't think as well. Look happy, confident, as if you can help them solve a problem. If you don't feel that way, pretend that you do. The old saying, "Fake it till you make it," really works. Shakespeare said,

"Assume a virtue if you have it not." If you pretend you are cheerful and self-assured, you will soon begin to feel it. The reverse is not true. Sitting around waiting to feel great before a speech doesn't usually happen. Everyone is nervous. They just go ahead anyway. They learn to channel the nervousness into an energetic delivery.

Wear professional clothes. A dark blue or gray suit with light shirt, striped, paisley, or club tie is good for men. Women should wear a suit or tailored dress without low cut necklines or skirts too short.

After you've written the speech and considered these do's and don'ts—PRACTICE. The more you sweat ahead of time, the less you sweat on stage. Practice in front of a mirror; in front of a friend who will give you honest feedback; or, best of all, in front of a video camera. Record yourself, watch it, and record again until you are pleased with your performance.

Pulling Teams Together-Meetings

No matter what the topic of the meeting you are having, people are worrying about three things according to William Shultz—inclusion, control, and affection. Inclusion deals with issues of acceptance. Will I be liked? How can I get to know these people? Will I let them know me? Control deals with the issue of power. Will I be listened to? Will I be able to get others to do some of what I want them to? What will I have to do to be a part of this group? Affection concerns how much group members care for each other. Do I care about others in this group, and am I willing to show it? Do they care about me, and will they show it?[10]

As the leader, how do you deal with these issues?

◆ **Inclusion**

Be sure each person speaks sometime during the meeting—the sooner the better. If they speak at the beginning of the meeting, they will usually feel included and pay closer attention. You can have people first write and then tell what they had to go through to get to the meeting or what task they left to come to the meeting. If it's a group of people who do not know each other, have them introduce themselves and then tell something about themselves.

◆ **Control**

If it is a small group, you need ideas from everyone at the meeting. Otherwise there was no reason to call them together. You will always have some extroverts and some introverts. Extroverts want to talk immediately and at length. Introverts want to have time to think before they speak. Because extroverts want to jump on a topic after you have barely finished laying it out and talk a lot as they figure out what they really think about a topic by sorting out the ideas aloud, you, as the leader, must exert some control over the meeting and provide an opportunity for each type to contribute valuable ideas. If you have everyone write on a topic for the first three minutes after it is brought up, the introverts have the quiet time needed to collect their thoughts. The extroverts have been forced to wait just three minutes, and then you can feel free to call on everyone to contribute his or her thoughts.

Do not let talkers dominate the meeting. If someone attacks someone, try to move in and stop it. You might say, "I don't think this criticism is constructive. Do you have a suggestion of a change we can make?"

◆ **Affection**

Showing affection may or may not be appropriate for your group. Members of some groups hug each other. In other groups, affection is shown by allowing talk about some personal concerns in addition to tending to business. The group may meet for coffee. If group members sense that others care about them, they are more productive, more willing to come to the meetings.

Long before a meeting begins, envision likely questions and problems so you can deal with them. Use the process recommended in the book, *The Inner Game of Tennis*. Just as you would visualize the correct tennis shot, "Visualize your meeting in advance. Picture the perfect attitude of the group, the perfect location, the perfect proposal, the perfect discussion, the perfect argument. Visualize the perfect response to the difficult participant. Visualize the perfect meeting and then make the necessary preparations to make that vision a reality."[11]

Try saying and picturing in your mind, "I will run a productive meeting where all the agenda topics are discussed and decided upon. People will cooperate." If you keep seeing it happen, it has a much better chance of happening than if you constantly ruminate about how Dr. Adams is going to negatively filibuster any changes that are suggested. Go talk to Dr. Adams ahead of time and try to win him over to your side, even if it requires giving him something he wants in order to get something you want.

If you know you cannot win over a dissenter, consider changing your plans. "'If I have something on the agenda that is really important to me, I always know where the votes are before I go into that meeting,' says lawyer and investment banker Peter Kelly. By doing this, you can make a judgment to move ahead on your item, to do a little extra homework, or to take it off the agenda if your count shows you can't win."[12]

Conflict-Confrontation-Anger

Knowing who to confront, when to confront, what to say, and how to say it is no simple task. Most people dread it. Don't expect that you won't. Even if you polish your technique, you still may procrastinate and have butterflies in your stomach when it comes time to do it. Some people report such extreme physical reactions as diarrhea, nausea, palpitating heart, and sweaty palms.

However, I have met a few physicians who truly seem to crave power, thrive on angry confrontation, and feel the joy of the kill when humiliating others with emotional outbursts. I suspect some of them went into medicine with a desire for power that would allow them to behave badly. Before the health care scene dramatically began to change in the late '80s and '90s, they could get by with such behavior for an entire career. With increased competition, some organizations are saying, "You simply cannot behave that way anymore. If you do, you will lose your job." "Problem employees who are not dealt with fairly and promptly will produce avoidable problems, demonstrate to others that poor behavior is okay, and subvert your management authority."[13]

The word confrontation usually has a negative connotation for most people. Try to switch your thinking to, "It is important that I learn to ask for what I want. Others should not be forced to read my mind."

Neither an angry voice nor a weak voice are effective in confrontation. Some people propel themselves into a confrontation with the use of anger. They usually meet with open rebellion or subversive behavior that undermines what they are trying to get accomplished. They tell people what to do, but somehow the projects are sabotaged. An anesthesiologist screams, "How many times have I told you this is not the proper set up for someone with cardiac problems?" The technicians get even with the physician by continuing to not set up properly and watching him explode.

Others ask for what they want with such a weak tone of voice and weak words that people do not take them seriously. "Would you mind not coming late for your shift?" A better way to say it is, "I have to stay late when you don't show up on time for your shift. I need to pick up my children. Please be on time."

Find an appropriate place for the confrontation. The hall will not do. "When the opportunity arises to compliment individuals for success and, even more important, for team success, a manager must do it well and let others in the organizations know about it. When it is necessary to correct, counsel, or admonish someone for any reason, it must be in private."[13]

Use a calm, firm voice with eye contact. Don't repeat your message in the beginning. Sometimes we deliver the message and then, either because we are nervous or we think the listener is ignoring us, we say it again and again. If you ramble on and repeat yourself, people discount you and tune you out. Say your major points and then wait for a reaction. It is not your job to try to make the other person comfortable by filling the air space with words. Also, you cannot afford the leisure of making yourself comfortable with constant chatter. Let there be silence or let the person blow up and just watch calmly. If the person explodes, let them blow. Do not become overly defensive. Stick to your major points.

If you are confronting someone about unacceptable behavior and you are met with much resistance and denial, you may have to repeat the message. Example: "Throwing instruments is unacceptable behavior in our organization." Becoming a broken record and repeating the message after you've listened to much denial is very different from saying the same message two or three different ways when you are beginning the conversation. The former shows firm conviction. The latter indicates nervousness and unsureness.

Discuss no more than three concerns in a confrontation—one is better. If you bring up too many issues you weaken your position. You cannot solve 20 years of irritation in one encounter. Don't bring up what happened in 1975. The more you confront things as they come up, the less you'll need to deal with all past hurts on the few occasions when you get the courage to say something.

You have a right to ask for what you want. You may not always get it, but, in this country, you can ask for it.

You do *not* have a right to yell for what you want and humiliate others with sarcasm in the process. Some of you may be thinking, "Oh, yes I do." If so, I encourage you to sit down and think about your relationships. Are the people who work with and for you cooperative? Are your patients leaving? Do your family members look forward to your coming home at night?

You also have a right to change how you behave in the relationship if you do not get what you want. For example, if family members will not pick up their own clothes after you have repeatedly asked them to, you can stop washing them. If physicians will not keep their charts up to date, you can intercept them as they enter the hospital to have charts completed.

Try not to use the big emotions of anger and tears in a confrontation. Some people use anger to try to get what they want; others use tears. Neither is very effective. People feel threatened, frightened, or repulsed by a show of uncontrolled emotion. However, if these emotions occur in others, try to remain calm and strong and not let them throw you off balance.

If you need to have an important confrontation or you have had an interaction that didn't go well, here's a process that may help you confront the person.

- Write out what you want to say or wish you had said and write how angry you are. Let all your emotions spill onto the page. Cuss them. Hold nothing back, but don't show this to anyone.
- Go for a 30-minute walk.
- Write again what you want to say. This time you'll find you don't need to say as many of the nasty things. Come up with three major points you want to make when you actually talk to the person.

1. Explain your view of the situation.

   I've gotten numerous complaints that you are yelling at co-workers and at times are even rude to patients. I've talked to you about this twice in the past six months. You do better for several weeks and then begin the same old behavior.

2. Tell what you want.

   This has to stop. I want you to get help to try to alleviate your anger and learn some better ways to communicate.

3. Say what will happen if you do not get it.

   If this continues, you will lose your job.

You may not always say the third point, but it is important for you to know. It gives you a sense of power, and people can detect it when you have it. When my children were small, and I was feeling exhausted, they would misbehave, because they sensed and probably feared weakness in me. Sometimes, I went across the street to complain to a neighbor who would help me come up with a plan. I'd walk back in the house with a strong countenance and a game plan. The children would take one look, see that the power was back, and shape up. Many times, I never had to do a thing. They seemed to be able to sniff the power in the air. The same is true for adults. If you look meek or unnecessarily mean, you probably will get noncooperation or rebellion. Find that middle ground that is firm but reasonable.

As a back-up plan, you need to know ahead of time what you are going to do if the person will not meet you half way on at least some of the points. You may not use this bargaining chip, but you need to have it in your mental pocket. People can sense power and they can sense weakness. If you have the back-up plan, the room is filled with power.

If you have no bargaining chip, don't keep trying to make the person change if you know he or she won't. Don't keep whining that you wish they would behave better. Every time you beg, you lose self-esteem and feel more humiliated.

In the '60s and '70s, much was written about the value of venting when you were angry. The advice was to really let the people know who have wronged you. I disagree. Few situations are improved with loud expressions of anger. Usually they just get hotter. Dr. Pierce Howard, in *The Owner's Manual for the Brain*, says, "The emotion of angry hostility places us in a double-bind: both holding it in and venting it are bad for the heart and the immune system. The secret to dealing with anger is to express it without getting angry. Get it out, deal with it, and get over it."[14]

Anger is a physical phenomenon as well as a mental one. You will feel it somewhere in your body—clinched fists, knots in your stomach, gritted teeth, tight neck, somewhere—because adrenaline is rushing through your system. You need to get it out of your body in a physical way, but there are many ways to do it besides screaming at the person who has angered you. Go for a run or a very fast walk. Play golf and pretend the ball is the offending person's head that you are slamming down the fairway. Write quickly without stopping, telling the person how rotten he or she is and what you want to do to him or her. (But don't let anyone see it.) You need to get the anger out of your system, but you don't want to dump it on the wrong person or even necessarily on the offending person.

There may be a few times when it is appropriate to get angry and let the person know it. Sometimes, people have to be matched with the same amount of force they are sending out. Not backing down on your position, looking mean, and raising your voice are essential to let the person know you can do it. I yelled only a few times when I was raising teenagers, and they speak of it still. They had to know I was capable of that much force. But you need to be careful not to do that often. Don't confront every issue just because you learn how to do it. Pretend you have five confrontation bullets, and they need to last you five years. Don't use them up too quickly or use them on small problems. Save them for big problems. Spilling juice on the kitchen floor is not a big problem; driving under the influence of alcohol is.

If you feel the occasion warrants an outburst and you simply must do it, do it once. If you don't get the results you want, next time confront in a calm, calculated manner with a plan for what you are going to do if the person does not meet your demands. Continuing to hysterically blow your top weakens your position, even though you may experience a temporary sense of power and a release of tension.

If you need courage to confront, try a technique employed by American Indians. They used "'power chants' as centering devices to keep their hearts open and their minds clear at times of great danger. Each Indian brave repeated a particular affirmation of courage over and over until it became so familiar it was second nature to him. That way, in a crisis he wouldn't have to think about it or try to remember the words of the chant. They would be right there at the tip of his tongue."[15]

If you need to calm down and not lose your temper, "call for a time out ('I'm too upset to talk about this anymore—I'd like to take a break and talk some more later.')."[16] Learning a relaxation technique can also help you gain control. Anger and relaxation cannot exist in the body at the same time. One rules out the other. After you have practiced the relaxation technique for at least three weeks, one or two deep breaths can help you control your reactions.

Take whichever approach will help you, but don't avoid the interaction too long. We are all different, and we must let each other know our needs in a calm, firm, effective manner.

Writing

Physician executives are called upon to write—memos, letters, reports, or articles. Memos stay inside the office and often travel up and down the hierarchical structure. Letters go outside the office and have to be dressed up a little better than memos. Reports often go to superiors. If you want any of them to be read by busy people, they must be short and sweet. The traditional academic style of writing will serve you well for clinical articles, but if you write for management journals, your style needs to be clear and less burdened with academic jargon.

Most of us get the necessary memos and letters written, even though we would rather do something else. But many people have said to me that they want to write an article or a book but just can't seem to get themselves to do it. Writing for publication lets people know who you are and what you think. It enhances your career, because people will consider you for specific jobs. It's a good networking technique, because it puts your name before people as an expert. I'll talk first about how to stop dreading the writing process so much, no matter what you need to write, and then about how to edit so you have a document you are proud of.

Frequently, when people have a writing project to do, they carry around with them a sense of gloom—I should do it, but I don't want to. They sharpen pencils, go to the bathroom, get another cup of coffee, clean out desk drawers that have been messy for months, go talk to someone at the water cooler—all tasks that seem urgent, certainly more important than putting the first word on the page.

If you want to stop procrastinating on writing projects, pick up a pen and write 10 minutes a day in a journal. A journal is whatever kind of paper you like. I'll describe it in more detail in Chapter 12.

Writing should be a two-part process—generating ideas and editing those ideas. Never do both at the same time. If you are writing along and can't decide which of two words to use in a sentence, write both of them down and keep going. "It's an unnecessary burden to try to think of words and also worry at the same time whether they are the right words."[17] If you stop to decide, the left hemisphere of your brain, which passes judgment on the quality of your work, wakes up and begins the censoring process. You have spent a fair amount of time lulling it into a rest mode by writing quickly without stopping. If you let it begin to work while you are brainstorming using the right hemisphere, the right side may stop sending ideas. All instructions for brainstorming in meetings say you must not judge anyone's ideas during the process of thinking of all the ideas you can come up with. The same is true when you are alone and brainstorming with pen and paper.

When you are having a difficult time making yourself write, start writing whether you feel like it or not. You may think you have no ideas at all on a subject, but, as Peter Elbow says about his own writing "you are making a serious error....You are mistaking lousy, stupid, second-rate, wrong, childish, foolish, worthless ideas for no ideas at all."[18] If you keep doing 10-minute writing exercises you will eventually find ideas you like. If you just sit, chew your pencil, wait for the ideas to come, they may never come at all. People use the term writer's block for this condition. It probably should be called writer's procrastination or writer's perfection. We all want great ideas to come on the first attempt, because it feels wonderful to be that brilliant. Occasionally, people do write great words on the first try, but it is rare. Also, we don't want to have to do the dreaded writing process a second time. When you decide to freewrite, all the pressure is off. You know it doesn't have to be good, so you just get started easier. People usually become hooked on this process the first time they experience writing something wonderful in the midst of lots of grumbling words complaining about the writing process.

It's not hard to write a journal entry if you give yourself permission for it to be lousy. If you will begin to pay your dues to the writing gods by writing anything that comes to mind everyday for a week, I assure you some good ideas will surprise you and turn up on the page in front of you almost as if you were taking dictation from some other-worldly source. "[A] person's best writing is often mixed up together with his worst. It all feels lousy to him as he's writing, but if he will let himself write it and come back later, he will find some parts of it are excellent. It's as though one's best words come wrapped in one's worst."[19] This is why you need to freewrite and put lots of words on paper—so you can find the good ones in the midst of much garbage.

You must put down enough words, whether good or bad, to get the writing process started. You exercise your hand and brain the same way an athlete trains for his or her sport. I find I rarely can skip the training process. If I have not been writing regularly in my journal, and I have a writing project due, it takes 5-10 days of 10-minute writing sessions to get back to producing sentences I like.

Once you have generated enough ideas and have written a draft of the paper, it is time to put on the hat of an editor and clean up the copy. "Every word omitted keeps another reader with you."[20] Editing is not as difficult if you have plenty of words to work with. You can pick the good and throw away the bad without worrying that there won't be enough left. Also, if you have generated the draft with a freewriting, devil-may-care attitude, you have not sacrificed so much to write the words, and you are more willing to cut.

"Editing means figuring out what you really mean to say, getting it clear in your head, getting it unified, getting it into an organized structure, and then getting it into the best words and throwing away the rest. It is crucial, but it is only the last step" in the writing process.[21] I've found if I read a draft the first thing in the morning for about five days, I'll edit more easily. Somehow I see things in the morning that I'll let slip later in the day.

Instead of trying to worry about all the rules of usage and grammar; I've picked a few that deal with how to be concise.

- **Avoid needless repetition**. It is fine to use the same word over and over when you are generating thoughts. As a matter of fact, the subconscious seems to send us messages that way. Often, a first draft of a paper will have a word repeated 5 to 10 times. When you are editing, circle all the repeated words and try to eliminate most of them, unless you are repeating the word to emphasize its importance or changing the word would confuse the reader. Examples:

  Too much repetition: Businesses want to decorate their offices with low-maintenance plants. Philodendrons and scheffleras are some low-maintenance plants. These plants are inexpensive.

  Improved: Businesses want to decorate their offices with inexpensive, low-maintenance plants, such as philodendrons and scheffleras.

- **Avoid redundancy.** Being redundant means that you write the same idea a second time, but use different words. End result, final conclusion, personal opinion, and unexpected surprise are examples of redundancy. Instead of the extra words used in a redundant phrase, cut to the simplest word. Clarity is better than stuffy sophistication. Examples:

advance reservations	reservations
basic necessities	needs
cease and desist	stop
each and every	all
first and foremost	first

- **Always use fewer words** rather than more words to express an idea. Examples:

in the event that	if
in order to	to
in the amount of	for
in view of the fact that	because

- **Use precise words** that convey a specific visual image rather than vague words. Examples:

nice house	brick house
pickup	Dodge wide cab
car	Jaguar

- **Choose strong verbs** rather than verbs hidden in many words. Examples:

make application to	apply
give assistance	help
make a decision	decide

- **Avoid jargon.** Jargon, in its broadest definition, is any language that is hard to understand. Sometimes it acts as a shield for those who don't have much to say. It can be specialized vocabulary that a particular group of people understand. Teenagers find a different set of words every two or three years that, they hope, will confuse their parents. Accountants, chemists, bankers, doctors, and others have their special terms that must be defined when they are working with the general public.

  Often jargon is phony, inflated, and uselessly complex language. A client told me once, "If I speak and write so others understand me, they will steal my job." I think jargon hurts you more than it might help you keep your job. People get angry if you use difficult words without explaining their meaning. They put your memos in the trash and do not do what you have asked them to do.

  The passage below from *Moby Dick* has lost its clarity and beauty through the addition of jargon.[22]

The Original

Call me Ishmael. Some years ago—never mind how long precisely—having little or no money in my purse and nothing in particular to interest me on shore, I thought I would sail about a little and see the water part of the world.

Jargon Added

You may identify me by the nomenclature of Ishmael. At a point in time several years previous to the current temporal zone—the precise number of which is extraneous information—devoid of sufficient monetary resources and lacking physical and/or psychical stimuli within the confines of my sphere of activity on land, I initiated several thought processes and concluded that I would commandeer a vessel of navigation with which to explore the aquatic component of this planet.

- **Eliminate overused words.** Overworked expressions make a reader switch from paying attention to your message to being irritated that you are saying the same old thing. "The bottom line," "the whole nine yards," and "I need your input" are phrases that need a few years' rest.

  If you can finish the following statements, they have probably been overused. Try filling in the blanks.[23]

  It has come to our ____________________________

  Please call at your earliest________________________

  We regret to _______________________________

  If you have additional questions, feel________________

  Enclosed _________________________________

- **Use the active voice** unless you have a specific reason not to. In the active voice, the subject performs the action of the verb and appears in the first part of the sentence.

  Example: The recruiting staff made three visits.

  Using the passive voice reverses the order of the nouns in the sentence and adds a form of "to be" (is, am, are, was, were, be, being, been) to the verb.

  Example: Three visits were made by the recruiting staff.

  Using the passive voice adds unnecessary words to a sentence and robs the verb of its straightforward power. There are times when the passive voice is appropriate. Perhaps you don't want to tell who is doing what. Example: "Valuable resources are being wasted."[24] However, most of us use it too often and weaken our messages. Use the active voice as much as possible.

  Examples:

An appointment can be made for you.	Passive voice
I can make an appointment for you.	Active voice
The new design was spoken about by Dr. Johnson.	Passive voice
Dr. Johnson spoke about the new design.	Active voice

When you are generating ideas, you need a carefree, relaxed feeling about your writing. Whatever pops in your head goes down on the page. When you edit, you use a critical eye and cut everything away but the straightforward information. If I need to edit, sometimes I will go to my flower bed and pull weeds to get me in the proper frame of mind. Editing is an absolutely essential part of writing, because no one wants to read all the aimless rambling that a human brain is capable of producing, but do not cause that editing shift to happen in the early stages of producing ideas. Once you have a good quantity of words on the page, you'll enjoy arranging them in a pleasing way. But if you have a blank page in front of you and let yourself think like an editor, you'll probably experience the overriding fear that there are no words in you. You'll have plenty of words when you sit down to write if they don't have to be perfect when they are first born.

References

1. Frank, M. *How to Get Your Point Across in 30 Seconds—or Less.* New York, N.Y.: Simon and Schuster, 1986, P. 15.
2. Ailes, R., with Kraushar, J. *You Are The Message.* Homewood, Ill.: Dow Jones-lrwin, 1988, p. 39.
3. Bethel, S. *Making a Difference.12 Qualities That Make You a Leader.* New York, N.Y.: Berkley Books, 1990, p.205.
4. Robert Jamplis, President and CEO, Palo Alto Medical Foundation, personal communication, Feb. 1995.
5. Peters, R. *When Physicians Fail as Managers.* Tampa, Fla.: American College of Physician Executives, 1994, p. 28.
6. Ailes, R., *op. cit.*, p. 52.
7. Wonder, J., and Donovan, P. *The Flexibility Factor.* New York, N.Y.: Ballantine Books, 1989, pp. 216-7.
8. Alexander, J. *Dare to Change.* New York, N.Y.: A Signet Book, New American Library, 1984, p. 138
9. Swets, P. *The Art of Talking So That People Will Listen.* Englewood Cliffs, N.J.: Prentice-Hall. Inc., 1983, p. 59.
10. Turner, N. *Effective Leadership in Small Groups.* Valley Forge, Pa.: Judson Press, 1977, pp. 17-9.
11. Kieffer, G. *The Strategy of Meetings.* New York, N.Y.: Simon and Schuster, 1988, p. 157.
12. *Ibid.,* p. 156.
13. Harris, C. "Physicians in Managed Care: Middle Management." In *Physicians in Managed Care: A Career Guide.* Tampa, Fla.: American College of Physician Executives, 1994, p. 88.
14. Howard, P. *The Owner's Manual for the Brain.* Austin, Tex.: Leornian Press—A Bard and Stephen Book, 1994, p. 153.
15. Arapakis, M. *Softpower.* New York, N.Y.: Warner Books, 1990, p. 151.
16. *Ibid.*, p. 152.

17. Elbow, P. *Writing Without Teachers*. London, England: Oxford University Press, 1973, p. 5.

18. *Ibid.*, p. 62.

19. *Ibid.*, p. 69.

20. *Ibid.*, p. 41.

21. *Ibid.*, p. 38.

22. Kolin, P. *Successful Writing at Work*. Lexington, Mass.: D. C. Heath and Company, 1986. (Originally appeared in Brown Alumni Monthly, Feb. 1981.)

23. Brill, L. *Business Writing Quick and Easy*, 2nd Edition. New York, N.Y.: American Management Association, 1989, p. 83.

24. Fielden, J. "What Do You Mean You Don't Like My Style?" *Harvard Business Review* 60(3):128-36, May-June 1982.

Other Reading

Lucas, S. *The Art of Public Speaking*. New York, N.Y.: Random House, 1986.

Chapter Seven

Networking—Getting to Know More People

One of the first and often the most difficult tasks for job seekers is to increase the size of their networks—the number of people they know. You need to get to know more people than you know now. Most people get a job because they know someone who knows someone that led to the position. People have to know who you are and what you can do in order to recommend you for a job. They need to see you tackling problems and working with people. I've known a few people who didn't have all the experience that the company wished that they had, but someone knew them and thought they had the qualities it would take to do the job. In this time of lessened job security, networking should be an ongoing process, something you are always doing, so that when you need a new position, you have people you already know that you can contact.

"Networking, which in the broadest sense is the maintaining of active friendships with your professional colleagues, helps you to stay current with developments in health care across the country."[1] "Stephen Rosen, an astrophysicist and career counselor who works with professionals from the former Soviet Union, tells his clients unfamiliar with the American business culture to 'network or not work.' It's that simple."[2]

Networking comes easily for some people, usually those who are naturally gregarious. They heartily greet everyone they encounter, ask them probing questions, talk about their accomplishments, and come away knowing the person's name and several memorable facts about them. Other people cringe at intruding on someone's private space, resist asking seemingly nosy questions, feel that boasting is offensive, and don't mind that they cannot remember the name of the person they just talked to. Even though it is difficult for some, networking is an essential part of the job search.

"Some people have said, 'I know everyone in my hospital, but I don't belong to any outside associations, and I don't go to lunch with people from other hospitals and other facilities. I just kind of like my own group.' The job search will be much more difficult if you don't have a broad network."[3]

Sometimes people have felt that they should not get jobs through connections—almost as if that was cheating. If they were good enough, they could get the job all by themselves. That's just not the way it usually happens, so you must face that you have to play the game because it's the only one in town. Another prevalent attitude is that networking is using people. If you return the favor somehow, someday, it's not using; it's what we all need—help from each other.

"Physicians are not used to networking. They are used to talking to people that they were in medical school with, but they don't know how to take it to the next step—talking to that person in order to get a referral to a stranger that they don't know."[4]

Gary Cohn in the *Wall Street Journal* says that management consultants and executive recruiters recommend, "DON'T BE SHY: The best way for an executive to gain entry to a company is through a personal recommendation, so pull out all the stops to get the word around you're available. Executives seeking upper-level jobs should generally seek help from upper-level contacts." Cohn also claims that 70 percent of jobs are landed because of personal contacts, 15 percent from placement agencies, 10 percent from direct mailings, and 5 percent from published openings.[5]

Sometimes you can even "create a job for yourself by contacting the appropriate person, explaining how you can satisfy that unmet need, and making an offer to work for them as a project manager or a consultant."[6]

To network you must increase your visibility—make speeches, write articles, serve on committees. Make phone calls, attend meetings and talk to people while you are there, send letters, send thank you notes, call people again, read journals for advertised positions, contact search firms. It's more work than most people want to do, but few people get to skip it.

Once you have accepted the fact that you must network, exactly how do you go about it? Make phone calls and then follow up with letters so people will have a written reminder of your conversation. If you want to move to the southeast, contact your medical school alumni office and find out which of your classmates live there. Then call them. Take the time to inquire about their lives before you immediately say what you want. Then, "Jan and I have always wanted to move back to your part of the country when the children were grown. I've been a medical director for an HMO here in Kansas for the past five years. Do you have HMOs in your town or a neighboring city? Do you know any doctors who work there that I could talk to?" And so on. You have a right to politely ask for information. You do not have a right to be pushy. The world out there does not owe you a contact just because you have gotten up, or have always had, the nerve to ask for one.

Attend meetings where people are gathered who are doing what you want to do. A 1988 article in *Medical Economics* lists organizations for groups of physicians interested in topics such as flying, art, law, ecology, handicapped physicians. They also list professional topics that gather physicians together in organizations, with our own heading the list.[7]

"Example 1: The American Academy of Medical Directors (former name of American College of Physician Executives) is "a forum for physicians with administrative, management, or leadership responsibilities.

Example 2: The Regulatory Affairs Professionals Society members are manufacturers of drugs, medical devices, biotechnology, cosmetics, food products, other items; lawyers, doctors, consultant, others in the regulated health care field also attend."

Other organizations you can join are American Association of Health Plans, Medical Group Management Association (MGMA), Healthcare Forum, American Hospital Association (AHA), American Group Practice Association (AGPA), or American Managed Care and Review Association (AMCRA). The *AHA Guide to the Health Care Field,* a reference book published annually, lists these organizations and others.[8]

Networking is not just begging for a job when you need one, although it is letting people know you are looking. It's ongoing, keeping up with people, staying in relationships, talking to people at meetings, calling occasionally to see how they are doing, writing a note of thanks when appropriate. Networking is also being visible. Without being obnoxious, let people see what you can do. Dress well, speak well. Volunteer to speak on something. Do a good job; give people valuable information. They'll remember you and think of you for a job. "Write for professional journals to create awareness or expertise. Get e-mail addresses of people, follow forums in the field, and communicate your knowledge."[9] People who find networking extremely difficult are sometimes more comfortable writing articles and giving speeches as a way to be visible to others. Also, "when you read a thought-provoking article in one of your professional journals, you should copy it and send it to people who might be interested in it."[10]

Even as they try diligently to increase their networks, some very bright people have trouble remembering names no matter what mnemonic games they try. One physician who had just learned a remembering trick said he met someone with the last name Dasher. He thought no problem—one of Santa's reindeer. He said that, over time, he called that man everything—Donner, Prancer, Vixen. Even if you have this problem, keep trying to remember. Be friendly, and maybe they will remember you. Whenever possible, write the name down and something about the person. Sometimes writing will imprint the name in your brain. Keep a file of the names, where you met, what they had on. Sometimes a bright color will stay with you as a reminder.

Before you go to a cocktail party or call someone on the phone, do your homework. Dale Carnegie described how thoroughly Theodore Roosevelt did his homework: "Whether his visitor was a cowboy or a Rough Rider, a New York politician or a diplomat, Roosevelt knew what to say....Whenever Roosevelt expected a visitor, he sat up late the night before, reading up on the subject in which he knew his guest was particularly interested. For Roosevelt knew, as all leaders know, that the royal road to a person's heart is to talk about the things he or she treasures most.[11] If you are planning to go to a cocktail party at an ACPE meeting, be sure you have read at least the current issue of *Physician Executive* or ideally the past several issues so you have possible topics of conversation. You may want to talk specifically to the author of an article who may be there. Many physicians write for the journal. Also read the *New England Journal of Medicine, Modern Healthcare,* and other health care management and medical publications for advertised openings. You may want to find someone from a particular organization at the meeting and ask them what it is like to work there.

Go through the list of attendees at a meeting when you arrive and see who is from an area where you would like to live and work. Find them at a session or cocktail party and talk to them about what they do. Don't just go up and tell them you are looking for a job. People are put off by that because they may not know of anything or they feel burdened by your request. "The worst strategy is to appear needy. If you are mentally carrying a begging bowl, you invite rejection....When meeting new people, your primary task is to project competence and confidence."[12] Get to know the person by asking questions and listening. Your turn to talk will come if you invest time in the relationship.

Also, before a social event, rehearse a two-sentence introduction, especially if making contacts is difficult for you. You should be able to tell who you are and what you do without hesitation, fumbling, or rambling. Example: "I am Barbara Linney, Director of Career Development for the American College of Physician Executives. I work with physicians who are thinking about making changes in their careers or who want to polish their communication skills."

"Networking is exchanging information, resources, and support in such a way that you build a relationship."[13] Without purpose, small talk becomes just pleasant schmoozing, chatting about the ball game, or commiserating about the weather. That may pass the time, but it's not networking.[14]

If you want information from someone in particular, try to find out something about the person ahead of time. Talk to someone else who knows him or her. Then you have a conversation opener. Example: "Jake mentioned that your organization was planning to open an office in Memphis. How soon do you think it will be before it is operational?"

When you meet people, ask them what they do, tell them what you do, and patiently let a friendship evolve. "[Y]ou should pose the most often asked question in the English language: 'What do you do for ABC?' It's not original, but it's 100 percent, red-white-and-blue normal and what people expect."[15] "People generally like to talk about themselves and their ambitions, frustrations, accomplishments. And they like to be helpful in ways that enable them to feel potent."[16] To get people to talk about themselves, ask questions such as, "The last time we were together you mentioned that you were going on a cruise. When did you get back? How was the trip?" Listen actively. Nod your head, say "uh huh," look interested. Make yourself be interested. People may know it if you are faking it too much.

As you listen to others, try to cue into ways that you could help them. They will often remember and return the favors. If someone helps you, immediately send a thank-you note. "When you're given a lead, a connection, or a valuable suggestion, the giver should immediately receive a handwritten thank-you note with a promise of reciprocal favors on demand."[17]

As you talk to others, don't be a whiner, a complainer, a naysayer all the time. No one needs another one of those in an organization.

After you've talked to someone for a while, introduce the person to someone else. Include some personal or professional information when introducing others so they have some topic to begin with. Example: "Robert, this is Julie Carlson. She just moved from Orlando to St. Louis to become the medical director for ABC Health Plan." Also, learn to tactfully break away from a conversation and meet others by introducing the other person to someone else and then moving away. You might say, "I'll call you next week" or "I have a few other people I need to talk to. I'll see you a little later."

Some logistical suggestions—at a cocktail party, hold your drink in your left hand so you can shake hands with your right hand. In today's society, anyone can offer the handshake first. Avoid messy food if you are truly trying to talk to people. Dripping ribs are just too difficult to manage. Carry fresh business cards in your pocket to offer when appropriate. People are offended if you are pushing business cards at everyone whether they ask for them or not, but you certainly want to have them on you. The easiest thing to do is have some loose ones in a pocket so you don't have to fumble for them.

"Don't attend one meeting, rush home, and assume you're on the road to a new job. Building useful relationships takes time....Speed the process by volunteering to work on a committee and by supplying your contacts with useful information."[17]

The following quote from *How to Fireproof Your Career* is valuable, not from the point of view of learning the labels but for showing the gradual building of relationships in the networking process: "*Acquaintances* are people you barely know. You bump into them in the cafeteria or at a Chamber of Commerce event, but you never see them again. *Associates* are people you see regularly because you have chosen to join in a group that brings you into contact with them at a professional association, an alumni club, or a volunteer activity. Over time, your associates experience you as someone who is energizing to be with, who can be counted on to come through with what he or she has promised, and who has valuable skills. *Actors* are the people on your list with whom you are actively exchanging valuable information and resources. You give them leads or tips.

They tell you about a resource or introduce you to someone you want to meet....Giving with no strings attached is the way to invite reciprocity. *Advocates* are people who go out of their way to find opportunities to refer and recommend you to others. *Allies* care about your success. These relationships are long-term and usually turn into friendships as allies see each other socially, as well as professionally. You won't have time to cultivate too many relationships to this level, so you much select these people carefully. CAUTION; You'll be labeled a 'nuisance networker' for sure if, out of enthusiasm or urgency, you violate the natural development of trust in a relationship...by trying to jump from acquaintance to advocate or ally."[18]

When you are considering a career change, you will not only attend meetings, but also want to talk to as many people as you can in all areas of your life. Make yourself contact at least five people a month. If you are in a hurry to make a change, the number will be higher. To jog your memory, here is a list of the kinds of people you can contact:

- Other physicians in your area
- Physicians in the area you would like to move to
- Members of committees on which you serve
- Members of your professional society
- Medical school and undergraduate classmates
- Military colleagues
- Friends
- Family
- Lawyers
- Accountants
- Competitors

"Don't forget to call your university placement office and alumni association. Look through your synagogue or church, social organizations, health club, and any other directories you have that contain names of people you know or who might conceivably believe they know or have heard of you."[19]

Also, as part of the networking process, you will want to contact physician executive search firms. Get to know the recruiters that deal regularly with the sectors of the health care industry of interest to you. You can find a list of reputable firms by reading the classified ads in the back of *Physician Executive*. Professional recruiters are excellent networkers and can help you find the job you want at no cost to you, as well as help you expand your network. These people will not immediately say to you that they will find you a job, because they work for the organization doing the hiring, not for the physician, but, if you tell them about yourself, they will keep you in mind as they try to fill their positions.

Figler uses an elaborate metaphor to describe the networking process: "Everyone has a friend who has a friend. Somewhere in that chain of friends, you are standing with your arms at your sides and your eyes closed. Now if you carefully open your eyes, reach out to the two friends waiting on either side, and grasp their hands firmly, you will feel the electricity of a personal contact network begin to course through your body. It will be stimulating, but not shocking. You will feel alive with the circuit of energy that comes from plugging into people networks. However, be aware that any time you drop your hands and close your eyes again, you have broken the connection. The life of the circuit depends on your ability to keep the switches open. I don't know how to help people who are asleep at the switch."[20]

Even if you are not literally holding the hands of people, you are making contact if you are talking to them. So get out there and talk—maybe more than you want to or are used to, keep talking and increase your network.

Make networking a way of life. "'I tried networking last Thursday and nothing happened,' says Janice in frustration. Of course not. It's a process, not an event. Sure, you have to begin by putting specific events on your calendar, but the goal is to make connecting a way of life. It takes at least six months to cultivate a bountiful network."[21]

When you are doing the hard work of a job search, "keep a list of activities you enjoy to reward yourself with when you complete your daily or weekly activities....Take a nap, a hot bath, ride your bike, garden, make a cup of tea and sit outside and read for half an hour."[22]

A networking quiz, taken from *How to Fireproof Your Career,* starts on page 97 of the work pages following this chapter. It is not meant to make you feel bad about what you don't do, but I think it is an excellent reminder of the possibilities of things you can do to increase your network. Take the time to go through it and then score your performance in networking. If you're like most of us, improvement will be called for. You might try picking one new activity a month to increase your network.

References

1. Tyler, J. *The Health Care Executive's Job Search.* Chicago, Ill.: Health Administration Press, 1994, p. 44.
2. *Ibid.*, p. 46.
3. Tiffan, W. "When Downsizing Points to You." Presentation at Perspectives in Medical Management, Chicago, Ill., May 1995.

4. Linney, B. "Bringing Reality to the Job Hunt Process." *Physician Executive* 22(1):53-5, Jan. 1996.

5. Cohn, G. "An Executive's Quest for a New Job Is a Lesson in Coolness and Strategy." *Wall Street Journal*, Nov. 19, 1985.

6. Marion, P. *Crisis Proof Your Career.* New York, N.Y.: Berkley Books, 1994, p. 167

7. Holoweiko, M. "Somewhere, There's an Organization for Every Doctor." *Medical Economics*, June 20, 1988, p. 170.

8. *AHA Guide to the Health Care Field.* Chicago, Ill.: American Hospital Association, published annually.

9. Donna Vavala, Health Communication Consultant, Odessa, Fla., personal communication, 1996.

10. Tyler, J., *op. cit.*, p. 45.

11. Carnegie, D. H*ow to Win Friends and Influence People.* New York, N.Y.: Pocket Books, 1981, p. 94.

12. Kennedy, M. *Get the Job You Want and the Money You're Worth.* Tampa, Fla.: American College of Physician Executives, 1995, p. 7.

13. Baber, A., and Waymon, L. *How to Fireproof Your Career. Survival Strategies for Volatile Times.* New York, N.Y.: Berkley Books, 1995, p. 201.

14. *Ibid.*, p. 208.

15. Kennedy, M., *op. cit.*, p. 6.

16. Figler, H. *The Complete Job Search Handbook.* New York, N.Y.: Henry Holt and Co., 1979, p. 190.

17. Kennedy, M., *op. cit.*, p. 8.

18. Baber, A., and Waymon, L., *op. cit.*, pp. 202-4.

19. Kennedy, M., *op. cit.*, p. 14.

21. Figler, H., *op. cit.*, p. 123.

22. Baber, A., and Waymon, L., *op. cit.*, p. 216.

23. Marion, P., *op. cit.*, p. 171.

Work Sheets

Networking Quiz*

Circle yes (Y) or no (N) for each of the following questions.

Y N 1. I see all those informal conversations at business and social events as opportunities to use my small talk skills to build relationships and expand my network.

Y N 2. I know at least 50 people well enough (professionally or in the community) to call and say, "Hi, this is [my name]," and they know who I am and what my capabilities are.

Y N 3. People in my network have referred me to at least 10 people who have given me some kind of career or personal information.

Y N 4. I'm comfortable calling friends of friends, and friends of friends of friends to seek information.

Y N 5. I belong to at least four professional or community organizations and am visibly active in them.

Y N 6. I read two trade journals or magazines in my field and two general news publications consistently.

Y N 7. I know people outside of my profession from activities, such as sports, PTA, or volunteer work.

Y N 8. I've taken at least one course or gone to one convention to help me stay current in my field or learn about a new field.

Y N 9. I stay in touch with people I knew and worked with at previous jobs.

Y N 10. I make a point of meeting people outside my organization, profession, or industry, and at all levels of the hierarchy.

Y N 11. At a social or business event, I'm comfortable with introductions and can remember the names of people I meet.

Y N 12. I introduce people to one another at business and social events.

Y N 13. When people ask, "What do you do?" I avoid long, confusing job titles and labels. Instead I tell what I do, simply and vividly, by giving an example of a recent project or success.

Y N 14. I let people know the kinds of problems I can solve, so that they can refer exactly the right kind of work challenges, job leads, or career information to me.

Y N 15. When I talk to people, I usually find up-to-date information on something of professional or personal interest to me.

Y N 16. I talk frequently with others for support, ideas, and resources.

Y N 17. I systematically network with people in my organization who work in other departments, other divisions, and other locations.

Y N 18. I have business cards and enjoy using conversation to look for ways to give or receive information or services so that exchanging cards is valuable and necessary.

Y N 19. I always find a good way to say, "Thank you," when someone gives me information or resources or a referral to someone they know.

Y N 20. I look for ways that my resources and information can help others fulfill their personal and professional goals.

Scoring yourself: Count how many times you circled Y, then analyze your score as follows:

1-10 Strengthen your career security as you learn the basics of networking. In the past, you may not have felt comfortable networking or may not have been convinced that networking could benefit you. However, you can learn how to do it, feel comfortable, and improve your on-the-job performance as well as your long-range career security.

11-14 You can give and get even more in your professional and personal networks as you develop your networking skills.

15-17 You have only a few gaps in your network.

18-20 Bravo! You're well on the way to experiencing the power of career security through networking.

* Adapted from Baber, A., and Waymon, L. *How to Fireproof Your Career. Survival Strategies for Volatile Times.* New York, N.Y.: Berkley Books, 1995, pp. 198-201.

Chapter Eight

Write a Powerful Résumé

Most of us put off writing or updating a résumé. It's sobering to review your work activities and put them in print. We are plagued with notions: Is it enough? Is that all there is? My whole life, and I'm supposed to put it on three pages—they must be crazy. Those considering career changes have to overcome the censoring voices and put together a résumé, not a curriculum vitae (CV).

"People don't read résumés. They skim them. If the first third of a résumé doesn't grab them, they toss it."[1] "While there is no consensus on how to write the perfect résumé, one thing is certain: you have just one minute to grab a potential employer's attention....[A] résumé is a marketing brochure and you are the product."[2]

A résumé is a short powerful document that showcases your accomplishments. It is a necessary document to use in a job search, but by itself it will not get you a job. "Warning! A résumé is merely a facilitation tool; it is a first step, not an end in itself. Some job seekers believe that the preparation of a good résumé is the most important part of their job search, but even the most stellar and professional résumé does not ensure success. In truth, a good interview is the most important....[A]s you embark on your job search, you will frequently be asked for your résumé. Without it, you cannot go to the next step, an interview."[3]

Randomly mailing résumés does not often get an interview for a high-level job. Word-of-mouth contact usually gets you the interview, but you must have a good-looking résumé to send before you get there. It must look as polished as your interview suit and give the employer valuable information about you.

A curriculum vitae, which many people have, is a long document—as long as it needs to be, because it tells all the places you have shown up for work, all your publications, education, everything you have done. We all need one to keep track of our professional lives, but it is not what you send a potential employer. Believe it or not people doing the hiring do not want to read all about you. They're busy or lazy or bored by too much information. If we become the ones doing the hiring, we don't want to read long ones either.

So write a short, powerful résumé to send to a potential employer—no more than three pages. That means you will have to pick and choose items from your curriculum vitae. Making it short forces you to put your best stuff down and leave out things you don't want to do again. Choose the activities that you have enjoyed doing in the past and would like to do more of in the future. Also, choose activities that are appropriate for the job you are applying for. If you want a management position, you would tell what you accomplished on a utilization review committee rather than a great discovery you made in your clinical practice.

An exercise that can help you make these decisions is to make a two-part list of things you really love to do and things you do well. "Examples of things you love to do in one column could be leading a meeting, making a plan, adding columns of figures, working with patients, mentoring a young doctor. When you picture this task, you have a feeling in your gut—I really like that. In the second column, list what you do well. You have gotten feedback from people consistently that you do mentor people well or you do plan well. You may have a list of 10 or 20 things, but it won't go on forever because one part of the list will eliminate some things."[1]

At the top of the first page of your résumé, type your full name, address, and home and office phone numbers (if it is all right for your office to know you are looking). Include zip code and area code. You do not want the employer to have to do the work of looking up that information. You provide all the information so they can easily get in touch with you.

Next, list your professional experience. It goes before education, because experience is the most important factor in getting a management position. You tell not only where you showed up for work and when (the items usually included in the CV), but also what you accomplished while you were there. People want to know most what you have been doing for the past three to five years, even though they want to read about all of your experience. If you have 20 years of experience, some information will have to be left out. When you choose items from your CV, most likely you will have to add information. True, you worked at St. Vincent's hospital from 1991 to 1995, but what did you do while you were there? Did you help lower costs in the emergency department? Tell how much. If you worked for a managed care facility, you might say: Developed four new satellite offices, recruited eight primary care physicians over a two-year period, and reduced the hospital utilization rate from 300 to 225 days per 1,000, which resulted in a first-time operational surplus for the plan.

Notice the numbers. People like to know that you have saved an organization money or increased its revenues, and they want to know how much and over what period. "[I]nclude the number of FTEs supervised, the number of departments reporting to you, the total amount of the budget, and the names of committees on which you served."[4] Use numbers to prove your general statements whenever you can.

Use strong active voice verbs, such as developed, recruited, reduced. An example of active voice is "John hit the ball." Passive voice is "The ball was hit by John." Stay away from the passive. Just as the name implies, it is not as powerful. Other action verbs: "chair, control, decrease, develop, direct, edit, establish, handle, implement, manage, negotiate, review, revise, supervise."[5] When applying for management positions, use some phrases, such as "led the team that," to show that you can manage people. Managers are not supposed to do everything themselves. They are supposed to help others to do.

You can use a chronological or functional format for your résumé. In a chronological résumé, you list what you've done in reverse order. For example, your most recent job from 1992 to the present is listed first under professional experience. Then you describe the position you had from 1986 to 1992 and so on, heading backwards. If you are running out of room, you may have to leave out some information from 15 years ago.

A functional résumé is helpful if you have been at the same place for the past 15 years. You can list the management functions you have performed in that one location in reverse chronological order. Examples: 1994-present, Chair of Strategic Planning Committee. 1992-1994 Chair of Hospital Utilization Review Committee.

"The further you go back in time, the more important it is to condense your responsibilities and accomplishments. The general rule: Condense heavily the descriptions of jobs held prior to the 10-year mark."[6]

Many recruiters will change the order and format of your résumé so the résumés of all the candidates they are submitting are uniform. But they will not do your work for you. You must present them a two to three-page résumé. I recommend that you list your professional management experience first, because that is what everyone is looking for. If that fills the bill, they will continue reading.

Education can be listed in the order that it happened or in reverse chronological order, whichever you prefer. Most of your education was in college and medical school, but people do notice if you have continuing management education if you are applying for a management position. The important concern for the education section is that you have the entry and completion date and the degree earned for each item. If it took you six years to finish college because you had to work to earn money, you need to mention that. Explain gaps of a year or longer, not months—that's getting too detailed.

What you include after work experience and education will be determined by how much room is left and what kind of position you are applying for. If you are applying for a management position, you would include publications on management topics, not your clinical publications. Many of those doing the hiring will look at a long list of clinical publications and say "So what—

you're not going to be practicing cardiology now." If you are applying to be Dean of a Medical School, you can include all your publications in a separate attachment, because publications are the badge of honor in academic circles.

Do include licensure and board certification. Most medical management positions require board certification. People ask, "Why, since I won't be doing internal medicine." It may be like a dog needing a pedigree to be a show dog, or it may be that other doctors you manage will have passed the boards, and they want to know that you made it through boot camp too. Fair or not, it most often is a requirement.

You can include honors (Alpha Omega Alpha, Phi Beta Kappa), languages (Spanish is impressive in Florida or the southern border states), special skills (computer literate), professional associations (American College of Physician Executives, American Academy of Pediatrics), or other information that you think is appropriate for the job you are applying for.

There is much debate about whether to include birthdate. It's your choice. Recruiters have told me they can figure it out whether you put it or not.

Do not put in the résumé why you are leaving your present position, your personal opinions, and salary history. The interview is the place to discuss such things. Don't list your references or say they are available upon request. Everyone already knows you will provide references, and you are wasting words if you tell them they are available. Also, do not give the names of your references until you have called each one of them and asked his or her permission. You want a reference to be prepared to talk about you, not caught off guard.

Once you have collected all the information you need for the résumé, you must think about how to dress up the finished product. People do pay attention to the color and thickness of the paper, the quality of the print. Just as you use fine linens on a dining table for important guests, you use fine quality paper to impress your potential employer. "Black type on white 24-lb. bond paper is still preferred. Use a 10-12 point (preferred) typeface in Times Roman or Helvetica and a laser printer."[7] Kennedy takes a firm stance on how résumés should be produced: "All correspondence should be done using a word processing program and should be printed on a letter-quality printer, such as laser or deskjet. Don't even think about typing. It tells the reader you're not computer-competent, and you will not be called for interviews. Computer competency is mandatory."[8]

The résumé often has to be changed from one prospective employer to another. You may find you want to highlight certain of your activities based on what the employer says it is looking for.

Some recruiters are faxing résumés to organizations. I don't recommend it. If you think you must fax a résumé, also immediately mail a good copy.

Be consistent in your résumé's layout. If you put professional experience, education, and other main headings in bold print, make them all the same. Don't bold print some and underline others. I know you will want to use all the space for your information, but having enough white space makes others want to read the document. Have top, bottom, and side margins and a space between major items.

No typing mistakes. "Have the nit-pickiest person you know proof it. A misspelling or grammatical error could be fatal. It's also inexcusable."[9] If your résumé has errors, people think you don't pay attention to details. Even with spell checkers on computers, it's almost impossible to catch all the typos yourself, because you've been working with the information so long you become blind to errors.

A résumé never leaves home without a cover letter, and every résumé sent out has a different cover letter. Otherwise, the person receiving it looks at it and thinks several possible thoughts: What's this? Why did I get it? Why should I read another résumé? It gets put in the trash can or is conveniently hidden under a pile so the recipient will not feel guilty about not reading it. The cover letter should tell briefly how you learned of the position, why you are sending your résumé, and when you will call to see if you can meet with the person. It is written on the same paper that the résumé is on. The cover letter is the last part in the writing process, and it is not written until you know exactly to whom you are sending the résumé.

"If you are sending your résumé to a search firm, you are probably one of 15 or 20 that they are looking at, because the search firm does the initial cut. Search firms are under no obligation to help you, because they are not in the business to find people jobs. They are in the business to be hired by companies to find people. How do they do it? By networking. Have a good cover letter that states what salary expectations you have, what you are looking for, and a few highlights from your career, but you don't need to repeat everything that's in your résumé. When they receive the résumé, someone will know what the current searches are. If it doesn't match any of the current searches, they put it aside. Don't expect to hear back from them unless they have an appropriate search under way. They are not going to call unless they have something hot."[1]

"The process of putting the résumé together is more helpful than the résumé itself. I would never urge anyone to use a résumé writing service. If you talk to someone who can ask you—What do you mean by this? Why is that an accomplishment? You say these things about your career, but I don't see any evidence of it—that is the help you need in a résumé."[1]

As much trouble as it is to write a résumé, you feel a sense of accomplishment when you finish. You get a concrete look at who you are and what you've done professionally. As you make plans for your future, it is important to examine your present and past to see if the direction you are heading in makes sense. Preparing a résumé allows you to place your life's accomplishments in order.

References

1. Tiffan, W. "When Downsizing Points to You." Presentation at ACPE Perspectives in Medical Management, Chicago, Ill., May 1995.
2. Marion, P. *Crisis Proof Your Career.* New York, N.Y.: Berkley Books, 1994, p. 169.
3. Tyler, J. *The Health Care Executive's Job Search.* Chicago, Ill.: Health Administration Press, 1994, p. 3.
4. *Ibid.,* p. 6.
5. *Ibid.,* p. 13.
6. *Ibid.,* p. 7.
7. Kennedy, M. *Get the Job You Want and the Money You're Worth.* Tampa, Fla.: American College of Physician Executives, 1995, p. 17.
8. *Ibid.,* p. 2.
9. *Ibid.,* p. 18.

SAMPLE RÉSUMÉS

Chronological Resume

William J. Anderson, M.D.

32 Parkway Drive
Dobbs Ferry, New York 10522

Office (203) 968-5555
Home (914) 693-5555

Physician executive in start-up, turnaround, and management of complex health care programs. Seventeen years experience with demonstrated strengths in leadership, operation, program development, negotiation, communication, and the bridging of clinical and business interests.

SUMMARY OF EXPERIENCE

Montefiore Medical Center, Bronx, NY 1985-present

A major academic medical center with 8,000 employees and annual revenue of $500 million. Multiple sites and programs throughout the Bronx, closely affiliated with Albert Einstein College of Medicine.

Vice President, Health Care Systems, 1986-present

Operating budget of $60 million with 1,100 employees. Managed a multispecialty medical practice, a home health agency, and prison health programs at Rikers Island and Spofford Juvenile Detention Center. Developed clinical programs and innovative business ventures for the Medical Center.

- Developed a high-technology home care joint venture. Generated over $1 million revenue and $250,000 profit in its first six months.
- Led efforts to develop program for 250,000-square-foot medical office building, joint venture imaging center, proprietary rehabilitation center, and center for sensory disorder. Collaborated with clinical department chairman, corporate management, and the board of directors.
- Negotiated 10 different HMO contracts, including bundled service, risk capitation, and fee-for-service arrangements.
- Successfully negotiated and implemented major service contracts with the City of New York and Empire Blue Cross totaling $45 million annually.
- Taught epidemiology and health care organization at Albert Einstein College of Medicine. Lectured nationally on changing health care delivery and managed care.

Director, Alternative Delivery Systems, 1985-1986

Operating budget of $15 million. Led the reorganization of the Montefiore Home Health Agency and prepared Montefiore for involvement in HMOs.

- Conceived the idea for and collaborated in development of a consortium of six academic medical centers that led to a metropolitan, areawide joint venture HMO.
- Organized, established, and managed an independent network of 175 Montefiore physicians to contract with HMOs, helping prepare the physicians for the new environment of cost containment. Generates over $2.5 million new annual revenue for Montefiore.

Westchester Community Health Plan, White Plains, NY 1980-1985

Independent, not-for-profit, staff model Health Maintenance Organization, acquired by Kaiser-Permanente Medical Care Program in 1985. Operating revenue $17 million, with 200 employees and 27,000 members.

Vice President and Medical Director

Chief medical officer and chief operating officer. Managed the delivery of comprehensive medical services. Accountable to the board of directors for quality assurance and utilization management.

- Accomplished financial turnaround by instituting utilization management techniques, improving service, applying sound personnel management principles, and implementing a state-of-the-art quality assurance program.
- Implemented performance-based compensation program for physicians, resulting in improved recruitment, retention, and morale.
- Developed and implemented a real-time information system for appointment scheduling, medical records, pharmacy, and utilization management.
- Managed clinical program transition during acquisition by Kaiser-Permanente.
- Practiced clinical pediatrics.

Community Health Plan of Suffolk, Inc., Suffolk, NY 1977-1980

Community-based, not-for-profit, staff-model HMO, with enrollment of 18,000.

Medical Director

Managed the development, start-up, and operation of clinical services. Accountable to the board of directors for quality assurance.

- Developed space program, staffing, clinical program, and control systems, and coordinated all hospital and specialty relationships.

- Practiced clinical pediatrics, and taught community health and medical ethics at SUNY at Stonybrook School of Medicine.

Montefiore Medical Center, Bronx, NY 1971-1977

Residency Program in Social Medicine, 1971-1974

Unique clinical training program focused on the education of graduate physicians in clinical medicine, community health, and change agentry.

Deputy Director, 1976-1977

Developed curriculum and supervised 40 graduate physicians in specialty tracks of internal medicine, pediatrics, and family medicine.

Resident in Pediatrics and Social Medicine, 1971-1974

Chief Resident, 1973-1974

United States Public Health Service 1972-1974

Commissioned officer in the National Health Service Corps, U.S. Public Health Service. Functioned as medical director and family physician in a federally funded neighborhood health center in Rock Island, IL. Honorable Discharge.

FACULTY APPOINTMENTS

1976-Present Assistant Professor of Epidemiology and Social Medicine, and Assistant Professor of Pediatrics, Albert Einstein College of Medicine

OTHER PROFESSIONAL ACTIVITIES

1981-Present Instructor and reviewer, National Committee for Quality Assurance

1983-1985 Executive Committee, Medical Directors' Division, Group Health Association of America (Secretary, 1984-85)

1983-1985 Member, National Advisory Committee for Health Care Management in the Workplace, Work in America Institute

EDUCATION

Columbus High School, Maplewood, NJ, Diploma 1963

University of Pennsylvania College of Arts and Sciences, Philadelphia, PA, B.A. 1963-1967 (American Civilization)

University of Virginia School of Medicine, Charlottesville, VA, M.D. 1967-1971

Residency Program in Social Medicine (Pediatrics) Montefiore Medical Center, Bronx, NY, 1971-1974 (Chief Resident 1973 - 1974)

CERTIFICATION

Diplomate, National Board of Medical Examiners, 1971

Diplomate, American Board of Pediatrics, 1974

Fellow, American Academy of Pediatrics, 1977

Fellow, American College of Physician Executives, 1983

Licensure: New York

PROFESSIONAL ASSOCIATIONS

American College of Physician Executives

Bromeen Social Research Group

American Academy of Pediatrics

Group Health Association of America

Functional Resume

Sharon A. Johnson, M. D.

Business Address
2350 Auburn Avenue
Cincinnati, Ohio 45219
(513) 241-2600

Home Address
10068 Leacrest Road
Cincinnati, Ohio 45215
(513) 771-4820

PROFESSIONAL EXPERIENCE

1985 to Present **President, Cardio-Thoracic Vascular Surgeons of Cincinnati, Inc.**

Managed large clinical practice (1,000 procedures) and teaching group of ten physicians. Facilitated relationship between physicians and five nurses, seven office personnel, and office manager all reporting to me. Developed and installed software program for retrieval of clinical data.

1992 to Present **Physicians Insurance Company of Ohio (PICO)**

Member, Board of Directors; Chairman, Audit Committee, formulated guidelines, initiated internal auditor system.

Member budget and finance, claims, underwriting and risk management committees.

President, Raven Development Co. (a real estate company subsidiary of PICO)

1978 to Present **American Medical Association**

Chairman, Liaison Committee on Medical Education (LCME) 1984, member of accreditation teams and chairman of team on four occasions.

Member, Council on Medical Education 1985 to present

Chairman, Ad Hoc Committee on Resident Supervision and Working Hours, responsible for writing guidelines and report with recommendation for revisions of requirements.

Chairman, Council on Continuing Physician Education 1981-82, developed programs for national meetings and organized the meetings.

1989 to 1992 **ChoiceCare (an IPA of over 120,000 members), Cincinnati, Ohio**

Founding member, Secretary and member of Executive Committee. Responsible for initial promotion and recruitment of over 1,000 physician members. Developed utilization guidelines resulting in reduction in length of stay from 8 to under 4 days. Negotiated with hospitals, physician subscribers, and industry. Directly involved in all corporate affairs, medical policy development, strategic planning, and board management of the HMO.

1979 to Present **Midwest Foundation for Medical Care, Cincinnati, Ohio**

Founding member, president (1980-1987)

Chairman, Utilization Review and Quality Assurance Committees (1979-1989). Responsible for recruiting over 1,000 physician members, promoting foundation to physicians and industry. Directed utilization review of nursing homes and hospitals; initiated preadmission certification; organized review nurses.

1980 to Present **Teaching/Attending Staff, Providence Hospital, Cincinnati, Ohio**

Member, Executive Committee

Director, Department of Surgery

Founder and Director, Vascular Laboratory (over 5,000 non-invasive studies)

1979 to Present **Teaching/Attending Staff, Good Samaritan Hospital, Cincinnati, Ohio**

Member, Executive Committee

Vice President, Executive Committee

Acting Chairman, Section of Thoracic Surgery

EDUCATION

1962 to 1966 St. Xavier High School, Cincinnati, Ohio
Graduate with honors

1966 to 1970	Xavier University, Cincinnati, Ohio B.S.
1970 to 1974	Stanford University Medical School, Stanford, California M.D.
1974 to 1975	City/County Hospital, San Francisco, California Rotating Internship
1975 to 1979	University of Cincinnati Medical Center, Cincinnati, Ohio General Surgery Residency Chief Administrative Resident 1977-1978 Chief Surgical Resident 1978-1979
1984 to 1985	Baylor University Medical Center, Dallas, Texas Cardio-Thoracic Surgery Fellowship

LICENSURE AND BOARD CERTIFICATION

Diplomate, American Board of Surgery
Diplomate, American Board of Thoracic Surgery
License: Ohio, Kentucky

ACADEMIC AFFILIATIONS

1980 to Present Associate Professor of Surgery, University of Cincinnati Medical Center, Cincinnati, Ohio

PROFESSIONAL ASSOCIATIONS

Society of Thoracic Surgeons
  Chairman, Government Relations Committee
American Association for Thoracic Surgery
  Chairman, Government Relations Committee
American College of Cardiology
International Society of Cardiovascular Surgeons
American College of Physician Executives
Ohio State Medical Association
  President, 1990-1991

DATE OF BIRTH

October 3, 1948

Cover Letter Example

782 Quinwood Dr.
Charlotte, NC 32821
August 8, 1996

Raymond E. Arnold, MD, MMM
Alpha Insurance Company
834 Lakeshore Ave.
St. Louis, MO 82346

Dear Dr. Arnold:

Dr. Edwin Moore told me at last week's American College of Physician Executive's meeting in Hilton Head that you are looking for someone in the Charlotte area who can help you recruit physicians for the HMO you will open in August.

As you can see from my attached resume, I have had considerable experience in the recruitment of physicians and in career planning with physicians. I believe that I could use my experience to help select qualified people who will be satisfied in an HMO environment.

I will call you in a week to see if I can meet with you when you are in town.

Sincerely,

George L. Manchester, MD

Work Sheets

Things I like to do:

Things I do well:

Chapter Nine

Interviewing for a Position

The interview may be the barrier that stands between you and your exciting new career. It's a time when we all want to seem intelligent, charming, eloquent, and full of dazzling stories of great achievements. But, in fact, many interviewees have experienced anxiety that left them stuttering over answers or chattering aimlessly trying to calm themselves. Some people who can do a job quite well do not get it because they do poorly in interviews. Preparing ahead of time and practicing the interview will give you the best chance of making a good first impression on an organization.

Prepare

You prepare ahead of time by doing research and learning all you can about your potential employer.

- Join professional societies or trade associations, go to the meetings, and talk to physician members. Ask them about the work climate in their organizations. Here are examples of questions you might ask.
  - —How are physician managers regarded by nonphysician executives?
  - —If you are interested in a national or regional organization, find out who makes the decisions. Will you have any power in the local organization, or will all final decisions be made somewhere else? Will that bother you? Will top management want to hear your innovative ideas?
  - —Does the organization have a history of frequently replacing top-level managers?
  - —Can you advance in the organization? If the organization has religious ties, does it matter if you go to that church or not?
  - —Does the medical director have power to make decisions, or is he or she just doing tasks that the doctors in the group do not want to do?
- Read magazines that discuss the kind of management job you want. Every trade association and professional society has its own journal. Examples of journals that discuss different kinds of management jobs:

Group Practice Journal (American Group Practice Association)
HMO Practice (The HMO Group)
Hospitals and Health Networks (American Hospital Association)
Modern Healthcare (Crain Communications)
Physician Executive (American College of Physician Executives)
American Medical News (American Medical Association)

- Call people you know in the organization. If you are interested in a management position and you know a cardiologist in a group, call the person and ask how he or she sees the role of the present physician executives. If calling people and asking them questions is difficult for you, write out everything you are going to say and have it by the phone. But talk in a voice that does not sound as if you are reading.

  "In the job search, you need to get used to the idea that people really rely on first impressions. Whatever you can do in the first minutes with somebody is important. Take time to script what you are going to say on a voice mail. Stand up and smile and have a script that is right to the point. So and so referred me to you, I've had x years doing such and such, and you have a mini commercial about yourself. When you listen to a voice mail message, you have a picture in your mind about what that person is like. The same is true when you are on the phone. All of that practicing and rehearsing is the kind of thing we do with people in our program and you need to get used to doing it in preparing yourself."[1]

  I have listened to voices on voice mail that were low, mumbly, rambling and made an immediate judgment that this person could not do the job. I know it may not be true, but others also make the same judgment and won't call you back or look at your résumé.

- Send a thank-you note to anyone who is helpful.

  Read anything that you can find about the organization or the particular area of health care that you will be interviewing for. "Your first, and probably most important, step to getting the job you want and the salary you're worth is research. There are two kinds of research: library and people....Please make friends with the reference room librarian and plan to cultivate and maintain this relationship indefinitely. Pick the library branch you frequent on the basis of this person's skills and helpfulness. If your local library isn't helpful, remember the Internet."[2]

  Call the public relations department and ask for the annual report and any brochures or publications that describe the organization. If it does not have a public relations department, ask the person who is scheduling the interview for you for any information he or she has on the organization.

- Ask for in-house newspapers and magazines that give the good news about the organization. Read the local newspaper to see if some negative news appears. "Look at important articles about that industry for the past 12-18 months. Remember, the most important information is how the industry/company has done" in the past five years.[3]

- Ask someone for an information interview. Using your network, find the name of someone in the organization you can talk to who might describe the work, personalities, or politics of the company.

  — Ask for 15-20 minutes of the person's time so they will know that you do not plan to tie them up for long.

  — Ask, "How are you?" Listen to the answer. If the person replies in a frantic way, "Busy, busy, busy," that tells you something about the organization or the work style that is needed to fill the job.

  — Tell the person you have three questions you would like to ask.

  Examples: How is the medical director viewed by top management? How is the organization doing financially? How do the doctors regard the medical director position?

  — Listen carefully as the person decides what other subjects to cover.

  Watching television one night I saw an example of great results from an information interview. Alec Guinness at 20 wanted to be an actor but didn't know how to go about it. After watching John Gielgud in the same play for three performances, Guinness called him and asked him how he could become an actor. Gielgud said you need an acting teacher. Guinness hired a teacher, and, a year later, Gielgud gave him his first part in Hamlet. In addition to working with an acting coach, Guinness had watched Hamlet 150 times. He had effectively sought information and then he did his homework.

During the Interview

During the interview you need to convey:

- How you can help the organization make or save money. Example: "As HMO medical director, I believe that I can help your organization reduce hospital utilization by 20 percent without sacrificing quality."

- Specific examples of your achievements in previous positions, each delivered in no more than a one-minute "minicase history" (focused on results, not activity). Example: "During my past two years as director of strategic planning and development, we opened four new satellite offices and developed two new departments in the main office."

- Knowledge of the industry (marketplace, products, personal contacts, inside and outside pressures). Example: "The contacts that I have made in my previous national organization as well as in two national professional societies have helped me to understand the competition in managed care."
- Knowledge of the potential employer's company (including its goals, challenges, history, and top management). Example: "I am aware that ABC HMO intends to be one of the largest managed care companies in the country in the next five years. I believe that my experience in development and contacts in the industry can help you realize your goal."

Potential Interview Questions

The following is a list of questions that are often asked in interviews. Take the time to fully write out answers to them before you go for the interview. You will not take your notes with you, but the information will be with you because you have so thoroughly thought it out.

- Tell me briefly what you've been doing since medical school.
- Why are you looking for a job?
- Why did you leave your last job?
- What were your major responsibilities in your last job?
- What is your greatest strength and your greatest weakness? (Try to couch the weakness in a positive light. Example: "I've been told that sometimes I'm too compassionate with subordinates." You can sometimes say your weakness is your strength taken too far. Example: "I'm very organized, but occasionally I'm so organized it slows me down. When that happens, I reassess the situation and speed things up.")
- What are your long- and short-term goals? Example of long-term—Become CEO of a health care organization. Example of short- term—Develop expertise in utilization management.
- What are the three greatest accomplishments in your career? Example: Led organization as it changed from being a local health care provider to a regional provider.
- What kind of contribution can you make to our company? Example: I believe I can organize and energize the medical staff so that its members would feel more supportive of the goals of the company.
- How do you react to criticism?
- Describe a time when you made a big mistake and how you handled it.
- Can you give me an example of how you have managed people in the past?

- How will your spouse feel about your taking this job, about relocating, about your work-related travel?
- Have you ever hired or fired someone?
- Why do you want a career in management?
- How would you deal with a physician who is not performing well?
- Describe your experience with utilization review and quality assurance.
- How might you bridge the communication gap between physicians and administrators?
- Can you describe a time when you analyzed a problem, set a goal, created strategies for solving the problem, implemented the plan, and evaluated the results?

"If you were unemployed for several months or even a year, be prepared to convince an interviewer that you weren't malingering or on a world tour. A gap is not an automatic knockout, because health care is in flux and some 40 percent of working adults have lost (and gained) jobs since 1990."[4]

"More organizations are doing telephone prescreening, serial interviews, group interviews, and reinterviews, but fewer are using stress interviews, which were hot a few years ago....About telephone prescreening....This is it—show time—the first interview. Stand up, gesture with your hands, and put enthusiasm and vitality into your voice. You can be out if you come across as dull on the phone."[5]

Practice the Interview

Get a video camera and read the answers to some of your interview preparation questions and take a good look at yourself. Kennedy says, "You need access to a VCR and a camera or to a camcorder for practice interviewing. If you haven't interviewed within the past 6 to 12 months, this is essential. Practice will increase your confidence if you have what you believe to be 'handicaps,' e.g., you've been fired, have been unemployed for more than three months, or are unlikely to receive a positive reference from your current boss."[6] "Record yourself answering every nasty, intimidating, or merely embarrassing question your helper can think up. Do this in one-minute segments and then play it back. In four sessions, you will be measurably improved. There is no coaching like video."[7]

If you need to change something, keep trying it in front of the camera until you are satisfied. Also look at a video of someone you admire and notice what they do with their hands, eyes, voice, face. Try to copy the person.

An interviewer is influenced as much by what you don't say as by what you do say. Facial expression communicates much more than you may realize. How do you hold your face? Do you look pleasant or grim? Relaxed or uptight? Do you sound confident but not arrogant or argumentative? Do you sit up straight, walk holding yourself up—not slouched over, looking meek. Do you have a firm handshake but not one that breaks knuckles? Do you have a sarcastic sneer more than you realize? A pleasant expression with an occasional smile conveys confidence.

When we are nervous, or even bored, we all exhibit certain comforting behaviors. We pat ourselves, scratch, shift in our seats, but watch how much you do them. I saw a female physician in a meeting comb her hair, get out a mirror and put on lipstick, take her shoe off and rub her foot, push to get the shoe back on her foot. This behavior should have stopped in public when a teacher called you on it in the eighth grade or when your mother hounded you about it until you gave it up around everyone but her. This behavior does not exude confidence. Don't do it, especially in an interview.

The sound of your voice is also important. Is it too soft or too loud? Do you always sound as if you are giving orders? Do you sound as if you could never give orders? Neither extreme is effective for management jobs. You need a confident, firm voice that can get forceful but that can also be soft when appropriate. If you are serious about this, you will have to ask some people what they think. Individual coaching is often quite helpful.

Most people are nervous during an interview, especially at the beginning. You can use some of that energy to help you perform well, but, if you are excessively nervous, you need to practice ways to relax. Purchase a relaxation tape and do it every day for three weeks. Your body will learn to relax and breathe slowly. If you get nervous during the actual interview, take a slow deep breath that is not noticeable, and you will find you will calm down. Expect some nervousness, and use the energy it provides to make you alert and energetic.

On the day of the interview, arrive 5-10 minutes early, wearing clothes appropriate for the job, the company, and the industry "culture." When in doubt, wear a conservative suit. For women, tailored suits with nothing low-cut at the neck and no extremely short skirts. For men, dark suits with ties that are not overly flashy. "Women: Your coat must be longer than your suit skirt. Men: Your coat must come below your knees. 'Suburban' coats for men (just above the knee) haven't been appropriate for any business since the '60s. You'd have to sneak it into the Salvation Army pickup box to get rid of it."[8]

During the interview sit up straight, speak clearly, and look at the interviewer. Don't fiddle with your hair, glasses, a pen, or clothing.

Don't chew gum in public unless you are a very discreet chewer. I've seen a few people who are able to move their mouths once every 5 minutes. I chew like a cow chewing her cud and pop it on every munch. A woman who took care of me as a child taught me to do this when I was five, and I felt enormously accomplished once I learned it. As an adult it has made chewing gum unacceptable behavior even in front of family members.

Don't appear arrogant or aggressive. If you argue with your interviewer, you probably will not get the job. Do not criticize former employees, bosses, or co-workers. If you do, the interviewer thinks you may do the same about him or her someday.

Be concise. Don't over explain. If in doubt, ask, "Is that what you wanted to know?" Ask questions at the appropriate time about your job responsibilities, management practices, the assignments of co-workers, and performance evaluations (how often, with whom, how done). Usually, near the end of the interview, you'll be asked if you have any questions. It's fine to have this list written down. "It is appropriate and sound practice to discuss advancement potential, job descriptions, and evaluation procedures during an employment interview."[9]

Let the employer bring up the issue of salary, but have in mind the lowest amount you would work for. Find out what people in similar positions are paid in that area of the country before you go to the interview so that you can know if the employer is being reasonable. Several organizations publish surveys of salary information for physician executives (American College of Physician Executives, Hay Group, Physician Executive Management Center, and Witt/Kieffer, Ford, Hadelman, and Lloyd).

Write a thank-you letter the day after the interview. Comment on something good that happened in the interview. Mention that you would like to work for the company. Reiterate or tell another reason why you think you can help the organization meet its goals. In the note you might say, "'After our discussion I'm more convinced than ever that XYZ and I would be a good fit'....Say that you'll be calling in the next few days to see if the organization has made a decision. Then call as you said you would. Talk to the secretary if the decision maker isn't there. Better still, ask for voice mail and leave a detailed message. Persistence pays off!"[10]

Kennedy recommends that you "call back every 10 days, probably every other Friday."[11] "Job hunters tend to see unreturned telephone calls as a sign of impending rejection rather than as carelessness, work overload, a snafu in the system, or simply the desire to put off a difficult decision. Impute no motive to unreturned calls. Call until you get through. Always talk to the secretary as if she were an ally and leave a voice mail message....Persistent, low-pressure wooing works best."[12] "If you can't reach any of the people you interviewed with, beginning with the prospective boss or personnel person, leave messages with their secretaries or voice mail. Explain that you're very interested in the job and that you're inquiring to see if a decision has been made or when one may be....don't apologize for calling or suggest that you're being a nuisance."[13] "Continue to check back regularly. Don't slack off on other targets. You can be rejected after six interviews."[14]

After the interview, how do you stand the waiting? You try to go on with your life, but every minute you are not doing a specific task your mind goes back like a homing pigeon. Did I get the job? Did I get the house? You wonder and worry. Is this the right thing to do? Is it fair to others in the family? What if it doesn't work out? What will we do?

How do you cope? As much as possible, turn your attention to other things while you wait in between the action steps. Keep telling people you are looking; contact other search firms. A retainer firm can only recommend you for one job at a time. Look at more than one job, more than one house, so you have options. This is very hard to do, because we tend to settle in on one thing we like and constantly ruminate about that one. "If you are serious about changing jobs and want to keep your momentum, not to mention your sanity and perspective, continue to interview right up until you accept an offer and give notice. If you don't, the importance of one near offer can be so magnified you will begin to believe that not getting the offer is the equivalent to career death. Even if you were 75/25 going in, you'll decide you must have this job. Don't put yourself under that kind of pressure."[15]

Plan on several interviews. "Certainly physicians who are getting ready to change from clinical careers to full-time management should probably interview for several positions before deciding on the right job, especially if they are going to have to make a geographic move. If a health care organization thinks enough of you to offer to pay your expenses to come for an initial interview, recruiters tell us that it is all right to go for that initial interview if you are more than 50 percent interested in the job. If you or your spouse is totally closed to living in that city or working for that organization, then it is not appropriate for you to interview for the position at the organization's expense. On the other hand, if you have doubts, but are open to the possibility, it is perfectly all right to go for that initial interview."[16]

Jennifer Grebenschikoff of the Physician Executive Management Center says, "Most health care organizations interview between three and five candidates in the first round of interviews. After that first round, the organization has usually narrowed the list either to one choice or possibly to two finalists, and, in that case, they will invite both finalists back for second interviews. Also, a physician should never take a job and the organization should never make a formal offer unless the spouse has had at least one visit to that new community."[17]

Employers want to hire enthusiastic people with good communication skills who will work hard. The interview is the place you can show them you have these qualities.

References

1. Tiffan, W. "When Downsizing Points to You." ACPE Perspectives in Medical Management, Chicago, Ill., May 1995.

2. Kennedy, M. *Get the Job You Want and the Money You're Worth.* Tampa, Fla.: American College of Physician Executives, 1995, p. 4.

3. *Ibid.,* p. 5.

4. *Ibid.,* p. 17.

5. *Ibid.,* p. 21.

6. *Ibid.,* p. 1.

7. *Ibid.,* p. 31.

8. *Ibid.,* p. 3.

9. Hartfield, J. In *Physicians in Managed Care. A Career Guide,* Bloomberg, M., and Mohlie, S., Editors. Tampa, Fla.: American College of Physician Executives, 1994, p. 77.

10. Kennedy, M., *op. cit.,* p. 25.

11. *Ibid.,* p. 37.

12. *Ibid.,* p. 36.

13. *Ibid.,* p. 35.

14. *Ibid.,* p. 24.

15. *Ibid.,* p. 35.

16. George Linney Jr., MD, FACPE, Vice President, Tyler and Company, personal communication, 1996.

17. Jennifer Grebenschikoff, Vice President, Physician Executive Management Center, personal communication, 1992.

Further Reading

Baxter, R., and Brashear, M. *Do-It-Yourself Career Kit.* Moraga, Calif.: Bridgewater Press, 1990.

Bolles, R. *The 1985 What Color Is Your Parachute?* Berkeley, Calif.: Ten Speed Press, 1985.

Figler, H. *The Complete Job-Search Handbook.* New York, N.Y.: Henry Holt and Company, 1979.

Steward, C., and Cash, W. *Interviewing Principles and Practices.* Dubuque, lowa: William. C. Brown Publishers, 1988.

Work Sheets

Potential interview questions:

Tell me briefly what you've been doing since medical school.

Why are you looking for a job?

Why did you leave your last job?

What were your major responsibilities in your last job?

What is your greatest strength and your greatest weakness? (Try to couch the weakness in a positive light. Example: I've been told that sometimes I'm too compassionate with subordinates.)

*Greatest strength*____

____

____

____

Greatest weakness ______________________________________

____

____

____

What are your long- and short-term goals? Example of long-term—Become CEO of a health care organization. Example of short-term—Develop expertise in utilization management.

Long-term goals ____

____

____

____

____

Short-term goals ____

____

____

____

What are the three greatest accomplishments in your career? Example: Led organization as it changed from being a local health care provider to a regional provider.

1. ____

   ____

2. ____

   ____

3. ____

   ____

What kind of contribution can you make to our company? Example: I believe I can organize and energize the medical staff so that its members would feel more supportive of the goals of the company.

How do you react to criticism?

Describe a time when you made a big mistake and how you handled it.

Can you give me an example of how you have managed people in the past?

How will your spouse feel about your taking this job, about relocating, about your work-related travel?

Have you ever hired or fired someone?

Why do you want a career in management?

How would you deal with a physician who is not performing well?

Describe your experience with utilization review and quality assurance.

How might you bridge the communication gap between physicians and administrators?

Can you describe a time when you analyzed a problem, set a goal, created strategies for solving the problem, implemented the plan, and evaluated the results?

Chapter Ten

Negotiating Your Salary

The idea of negotiation raises the anxiety level of all but a few people, those who thrive on the thrill of competitive bargaining. Most physicians I've met do not relish the process and view it as a type of conflict. "Most of us react to conflict the same way our ancient ancestors reacted to saber-toothed tigers appearing on the horizon. Our instinct is still 'fight or flight,' however much we have evolved in other areas. Our primitive urge is either to fight back and escalate the conflict, or to run away. This flight may mean actually leaving the room, or simply withdrawing emotionally. When you give in to either fight or flight, you lose control of the situation and are likely to feel either abusive or victimized."[1] Kennedy says, " Unless you're prepared to overcome a natural reluctance to make counteroffers (in a negotiation), your options are not just limited, they're nonexistent."[2] "[O]ne of the rules of the '90s is, 'Get the money up front.'"[3]

I interviewed Bettina Kilbourne, who was offered less than she wanted for her first physician executive job. She asked a friend who was a recruiter to coach her through the process. The recruiter said, "Remember, they can afford more than that." Kilbourne says, "Women have to be especially careful that they don't get sucked into trying to take care of everyone's needs and thinking, "Oh well, gosh. If they really don't have the budget, blah, blah, blah." In a negotiating situation, the "nurturing" approach is inappropriate. It doubly arms the person with whom you are negotiating salary and terms.

"Employment negotiations are complex not only because there are so many potential items to negotiate but also because you need to maintain a good relationship with your future employer during the process....Mutual respect needs to be maintained throughout the negotiating process. If something goes wrong at this stage, it could jeopardize the offer of employment or you could end up wishing you had never accepted the position."[4]

In order to curb the inclination to fight or flee, determine what you want before you get into an important negotiation. It is even better if you write down your desires. You will get clear on what you want much quicker and you will remember the points better when you talk to the other person. Try to stick with honestly saying to yourself what you want rather than veering off in all directions about what you should want.

"[Y]ou are negotiating not just a salary but a package, which may include such things as salary, bonus, vacation, educational leave, insurance (health, life, dental, disability are possibilities), flexible hours, child care or elder care leave, flexible benefit plans, retirement plans, and relocation packages."[4] Other benefits you might ask for are paying dues for one specialty society and one management association, car or allowance for a car if your job requires lots of travel, assistance with buying out a malpractice tail, and a severance package. A position with a relatively high salary and no benefits may not answer your needs, despite the attractive salary. On the other hand, if the benefits are very generous and fit your needs, you may be willing to take a somewhat lesser salary."[4]

You need to know what other people are getting paid for jobs similar to yours. This requires research. Several executive recruitment firms (the Physician Executive Management Center, Tampa, Florida; Witt/Kieffer, Ford, Hadelman and Lloyd, Oakbrook, Illinois; and Cejka and Company, St. Louis, Missouri, for instance) and national health care associations, (ACPE, American College of Healthcare Executives, and others) collect data on compensation for the professions they serve. In addition, health care periodicals, such as *Modern Healthcare* and *Hospitals and Health Networks,* have annual reports of compensation surveys. Kennedy recommends you also do your own survey. Call people and say, "'I need to get an idea of what your organization would (does) pay for that job; when I've finished my survey, I'll send you a copy.'...Also talk with headhunters, look at industry surveys, do a literature search at the library, network out of town. The key is to establish a defensible range. Be prepared to produce your documentation if asked."[5]

After you've become clear about your desires and you are meeting with a representative of the organization, do not announce those desires when you first encounter the other person. "After you know what you want, the next step is to find out what the other person wants....Don't guess, and don't assume. ASK."[6] It is important to pay attention carefully before it is your turn to present your wants. "When you...arrive at the negotiating event, you must discipline yourself to practice effective listening techniques. If you are carefully concentrating on what's going on, you can learn a great deal about the other side's feelings, motivation, and real needs."[7]

If you listen first, you will have a better chance of being heard when you speak. "People listen better, sooner, and longer when you speak to their needs first...but...research shows that people speak first to the other person's needs only three percent of the time....We usually speak first to our own needs because we are unclear about what we want and are trying to figure it out as we talk, or because we're secretly afraid we can't have it and we are trying to trick, overwhelm, or fast-talk others into giving it to us. The result is that people close down and are less receptive to what we say."[8] You will be able to listen carefully if you have done your research and written down what you want before the negotiation begins.

An organization that is interviewing you for a physician executive position might offer you a salary of $140,000 and the standard benefits of health, life, dental, and disability insurance, retirement, vacation, and CME time. You might want some additional benefits, such as car allowance, relocation costs, or tuition for an MBA.

After you have listened carefully to the other person's needs, it is essential to let them know you have heard them. Here is a possible opening for your part of the negotiation after you have listened well: "I am really pleased that you want me for this position, and I think that I could accept your base salary and benefits, even though they are lower than what I had hoped for, if you could give me...."

Try to have some logic to support what you want. Don't ask for an automobile allowance unless you are traveling for the company. If you park your car in the office lot from 8 a.m. to 6 p.m., don't expect a car allowance. Ask for financial assistance with obtaining an MBA if you feel that would enhance your value to the organization. You could ask for moving expenses or a signing bonus as a way to enhance the initial package and allow the organization to keep the base salary in line with other executive salaries.

"Train yourself to say, in every one of your negotiations, 'If everything goes wrong, will my life end?' If the answer to this question is no, teach yourself to say, 'Big deal, Who cares?' and 'So what?' Develop the attitude of caring—but not caring that much."[9]

"Employment contracts are an option in some companies, but most will not offer them. It is worth it to ask for one, but even if it is not offered, make sure that you get all your agreements in writing in an offer letter. This is critical and can be just as legally binding as an employment contract."[10] "Our best advice is not to resign your present job until you have this written offer. Too many colleagues have been caught without any job at all because they failed to take this simple and reasonable step....Remember, you can negotiate a reasonable contract for yourself if you arm yourself with information and get it all in writing."[11]

Negotiation That Went Well

The following is an example of how a physician negotiated to get a job and then continued to use negotiation skills when he was in the medical director position:

"I left pediatric practice in 1986 after being in practice for 30 years. I went to work for Prudential PruCare. I was the 51st person they interviewed for a statewide medical director position. I told them I wasn't interested in the job, and I wanted to be the last one interviewed. I knew nothing about managed care.

"I had lunch with them. I was honest with them. I said, 'Number one, I am not running away from pediatric practice. I'm thinking of a second career. I'm moving to something better. I love pediatrics. I could spend the rest of my life in it and be happy. I am going to something. I'm not running away.' That's the first point that I got across. The second point was that I was always an innovator. I demonstrated how I had had a full-time pediatric practice and basically was only in the office three days a week.

"They asked me, 'How do you think you would do in this job after practicing for 30 years? Do you think you could discipline physicians and do what's necessary?' I said, 'My wife and sons know me better than I know myself. I'm going to go home and ask them if I can do it.' They said, 'You're the kind of person we are looking for—one who has an open mind,' and they handed me a contract.

"I think they wanted to take a chance on somebody who had different ideas. I stayed with them for five or six years. I learned a lot. That's when I got involved in ACPE, because when I took the job, I knew nothing about management skills.

"I was their first full-time medical director in the entire country. I wasn't sure I wanted to give up pediatric practice, so I negotiated staying in practice and working full time with Prudential. At the beginning when I went to work for Prudential, I was dying to get back to my practice, but, as the years went by, I was dying to get back to Prudential. Two and a half years later, I closed my office.

"My wife loves to read ads. She read about a job opening in western Massachusetts. She said, 'I want to go to a craft show out there, and there is a small HMO that is advertising for somebody. Why don't you set up an interview so you can drive out there with me.' It was a small HMO—five or six years old—that I wasn't really interested in, so I decided I would negotiate like heck. They offered me a salary that was one and a half times what I was making at Prudential. And I said, 'No, that's not nearly enough.' They said, 'That's the highest we can go.' So I said, 'That's a four-day-a-week salary. I'll only work four days a week.' They said, 'That's fine. You can take off every Friday.'

"I found a gorgeous new home, which is why I took the job. I never could have afforded it in the Boston area. I like to do crafts, and I have a 72-foot workshop in the basement. A magnificent home that in the Boston area would have been millions of dollars, and here it was $360,000. I looked at the house, which has 44 windows, and I said I need money to put curtains on the windows. I negotiated for decorating costs. By then I figured I had a good deal.

"What I got as a bonus was that, because it was a young company, the senior management team had planned a supplementary retirement plan for themselves that was taxable at the end of the year but was based on average salary and the number of years until you were 65. They were getting 3 or 4 percent of their gross pay as a cash payment at the end of the year. This was in addition to their 401k. I came in at the age of 58 and had 7 years to retirement, so I get 20-25 percent of my total reimbursement each year as a cash payment.

"In negotiating a salary, if an organization wants somebody, they will be willing to pay. I never burned my bridges behind me. I always had a place to go back to, and I wasn't running away from my practice."

When I asked the physician how he learned to negotiate like that, he said, "I grew up in the depression. I was a street kid. My parents taught me if you don't ask you'll never get. The secret to negotiation to me is to make the interpersonal relationship with the people good and to give them what they want. You can't win anything by taking things away from people. You can win by giving things to people. This is how I got the doctors and everybody in the plan to be so productive. I never went in with a punitive attitude. I always went in with the attitude of giving them something extra, showing them why it would be in their best interest to do something rather than why it would be in their worst interest not to do something.

"I always negotiated by showing the person how they were getting the better part of the deal. In one of the doctor's offices, the secretaries at the end of the day would send patients to the emergency department instead of having them be seen by the doctor. This was a capitated plan. $250 for the emergency department visit. Nothing for the office. Big problem. I did two things to solve this problem. I'm good with computers. I found out that a way I could identify when this was happening was by comparing the ratio of office visits to specialty referrals. If there were very few office visits and a lot of specialty referrals, I knew the secretary was doing this at the end of the day. I called up the secretaries and said, 'Don't you like big bonuses at the end of the year? Your doctor gets bonuses for money that is not spent, and the people who go to the emergency department cost money. The bonus will be less, and you will get less money at the end of the year.' They started to get the patients into the office earlier. That helped a little bit.

"Then I turned it around the other way in talking with the doctors. The average doctor with a panel of 300 patients has 300 emergency department visits a year. Let's say that's what the average doctor in a specialty does. I made patient age and gender adjustments so one doctor couldn't claim having a sicker panel of patients than others. I explained costs to the plan and to the doctors. 'What we will do is open an account for you and we'll credit you with $50 times 300 visits, or $15,000. Every time one of your patients goes to the emergency department, justified or unjustified, we'll deduct $50 from that account and at the end of the year you will get the balance that's left in it.' The doctors said to me, 'You're fining us $50 every time we see a patient.' I said, 'No, I'm giving you $15,000. You're spending your own money. How you spend it is up to you.' Emergency department referrals dropped 25 percent immediately, and they stayed down. The next year, we took the average number of referrals and established a $12,000 credit per doctor. It dropped to $9,000 the next year. We are spending less and less for emergency department referrals because each year we renegotiate the credit. And the doctors are tickled pink. A punitive negotiation has been turned into a very positive one that gives them an incentive to do something.

Negotiation That Did Not Go Well

The following is an example of a negotiation that did not go well. I think you will see that, in some situations, all the negotiation techniques in the world won't work, because the power rests with the other side.

"I work in a pediatric intensive unit in a general hospital. I have accomplished quite a bit for the unit—utilization census improved over the past two years from 700 annual admissions to more than 900 admissions. Physician revenues improved from $700,000 to more than $1 million dollars. I felt, from administrative as well as financial aspects, that I had done a good job and deserved an increase in salary. I get straight salary with a potential bonus if we collect beyond a certain figure. I outlined all my accomplishments for the past two years and sent them to the COO. I didn't hear from him for over a month, so I sent another memo reminding him.

"He outlined a financial arrangement that a consultant had recommended. There is a 10 percent reduction of my salary if I perform to the best of my ability. If I don't perform to the best of my ability, there is a 40 percent reduction.

"The same thing was done to me two years ago. It was an unpleasant negotiation. We were in turmoil. We had an incompetent physician that I insisted be fired. They didn't want to put themselves in a position where they would be sued by this physician. When they refused to get rid of her, I walked out. I got a position at another institution and worked for one day, and then they faxed me in my hotel and said, 'Whatever your requirements, we will meet them. Please come back.' I came back. They forced her to resign and gave her four months' severance. Twenty-four hours before my contract expired, I got everything I needed. However, at that time I was in the driver's seat.

"Now the COO thinks he's got me in his grip. Then, I was the only intensivist left to take care of patients in the ICU. Whatever I asked for, I got. Now it's the other way around. I've been able to recruit two intensivists whose contracts are not due to be renewed for another year. The COO is in the driver's seat. He can now force me to accept the terms that he wanted me to accept two years ago. I'm in a bind, because I've indicated I'm not interested in moving anywhere else. I am happy with the hospital, and I've accomplished quite a bit—increased nursing staff, increased beds. The unit serves as a model for other units in the hospital. I feel we are finally moving in the right direction, and I don't want to just throw everything away and move.

"I had not seriously looked anywhere else until last week. I think they feel I don't have any other alternatives, so I've started looking to see what's available. I've gotten them to verbally agree to extend the arrangement through July."

This situation was not resolved when I interviewed the physician. My guess is there will not be a positive outcome from the physician's point of view. There were bad feelings between the parties from a previous negotiation, and the hospital was not desperate for the physician's services this time. Another physician said, "It's a question of supply and demand. If you are one of a hundred people who are lining up for a job and everybody looks about the same, your negotiating position is a lot less than if there are a 100 people and you are much more highly qualified than the others. In my case, a new position was created, and I fit the bill very nicely, so I had the power on my side. If you are really in demand, you can *almost* name your price, but you can't be greedy. If, on a scale of 1 to 10, you are perceived to be a 7, and you think you should be paid as a 10, it's not going to work. If you say you deserve the world, you lose credibility."

Some summary advice: If you are going to negotiate a salary, do it in person. And don't let the person you're negotiating with know you don't want to move. He or she needs to always think you have options.)

References

1. Anderson, K. *Getting What You Want. How to Reach Agreement and Resolve Conflict Every Time.* New York, N.Y.: Plume Books, 1994, p. 5.
2. Kennedy, M. *Get the Job You Want and the Money You're Worth.* Tampa, Fla.: American College of Physician Executives, 1995, p. 27.
3. *Ibid.,* p. 31.
4. Buyse, M., and Falcao-Blumenfeld, P. "Negotiating Contracts." *Journal of the American Medical Women's Association* 46(3):75,76,82, May-June 1991.
5. Kennedy, M., *op. cit.,* p. 28.
6. Anderson, K., *op. cit.,* p. 13.
7. Cohen, H. *You Can Negotiate Anything.* Secaucus, N.J.: Lyle Stuart Books, p. 106.
8. Anderson, K., *op. cit.,* p. 21.
9. Cohen, H., *op. cit.,* p. 88.
10. Buyse, M., and Falcao-Blumenfeld, P. *op. cit.* p. 75.
11. Buyse, M., and Falcao-Blumenfeld, P., *op. cit.,* p. 82.

Work Sheet

Minimally acceptable salary ________________________

Desired salary ________________________

Required benefits ________________________

Desired benefits ________________________

Chapter Eleven

What to Do When Fired

Organizations are merging. Managed care and capitation are spreading. Organizations are holding their executives responsible for profits and losses. These things are causing physician executives to lose their jobs. Hardworking, conscientious, charming, politically astute people are losing their jobs. How might you see it coming, and how can you cope with and move through the loss?

Here are some warning signs that you may be the victim of downsizing and some conditions that might increase your vulnerability[1]:

1. Others know you don't like what you do.
2. People stop listening to you. You are not included in meetings. You are not part of decision making.
3. You receive negative performance reviews.
4. You are not personally productive. You don't do anything new or creative.
5. You are failing to change, for instance are unwilling to learn to use new technology. People say that you refused to learn a new technique because you didn't agree with the change.
6. You aren't comfortable with a new culture.
7. You have poor communication skills—talk too much or too little.
8. You miss objectives set by you or your boss.
9. Economic conditions are negative. Census is going down. In a new organization created by acquisition or merger, only one CEO or medical director is needed. Under capitation, fewer people are needed to do the job.
10. You cost too much. Someone can be brought in at half the price to do the job.

"Because it's so traumatic, job loss is the third most severe loss people can suffer. In many ways, people's reactions to losing their jobs duplicate their reactions to the number one loss, death of a loved one, and the number two loss, divorce....Throughout the loss cycle, people report feeling a lack of control, increased stress, mounting anxiety, and moments of heart-stopping fear....Some people move quickly through the various stages after they have been laid off; others move slowly, taking as much as a year or more to complete the cycle; others move forward and then drop back to repeat a stage in a sort of two steps forward, one step back pattern.[2]

The following is a description of reactions people usually experience when they lose jobs. The list is not meant to imply that you must go through all these reactions in a prescribed order to get over the loss, but it is meant to remind you that, if you are experiencing some or all of these feelings, they are normal and expected. "If you know how people typically react to job loss, you can move more quickly through the stages that make it difficult to begin again."[3]

Shock

In this stage, occurring immediately after they are told they will be laid off, people are numb and unresponsive. They find it difficult to do anything, even to talk.

Denial

In this stage, a common reaction is disbelief. Some people, after they have been notified, race around trying to finish a project or a report as if they refuse to believe that their job has ended.

Anger

In this stage, people say things like, "They can't do this to me. I'll show them. I don't deserve this. Where's my lawyer?'" Typically, men exhibit more anger than women do. They sometimes deny their feelings of depression, guilt, and grief. Women deny and internalize their anger, turning it into depression, guilt, and grief. People who get in touch with all these feelings move through the cycle more quickly.

Bargaining

In this stage, people fantasize about steps they could have taken in the past to avoid being laid off. Round and round they go in their minds, like a hamster running a wheel.

Guilt

In this stage, people blame themselves for the loss of job. They are ashamed. They revisit in their minds every lapse or failure or rejection in their lives. The disappointments and hurts of a lifetime come rushing back into their minds.

Depression

In this stage, people question their value. "I'm no good. It's no wonder they don't want me." They gain or lose weight, sleep too much or too little, hide away, and hit bottom.

Grief

In this stage, people reflect on what they have lost and are sad. They mourn the loss. Even if they didn't love their jobs, they mourn the loss of the familiar.

Acceptance

In this stage, people begin to "get on with it." They say, "There's nothing I can do about it." They feel excitement about the future.

Involvement and Commitment

In this stage, people are ready to become involved with a new organization and to make a commitment to that organization, although it is often a different kind of work commitment than they have ever made in the past. They recognize that the greater your investment in your job, the more devastating it is to lose. They vow in the future to maintain a better balance between work and the rest of their lives."[4]

The following suggestions can sometimes help you move through the stages more quickly:

- "Keep a journal. A private log of your thoughts and feelings can help you get in touch with and sort through your emotions. Research indicates that people who keep journals not only move through the stages more quickly, but also find reemployment more quickly."[3]
- Tell your spouse. Even though your spouse will also be going through the loss cycle, you will both move through it more quickly if your spouse is not blaming and resentful.
- Talk to a friend about the emotional ups and downs. It is especially helpful if you can talk to people who have been through the experience.
- Talk to a professional counselor.

Two Real-Life Experiences

Following are interviews with two physician executives who experienced job loss. Details have been altered to protect the identity of the interviewees.

First Physician Executive

What position did you have?

I was Chief Medical Officer of a large tertiary hospital in the Northwest. I had been there a little over 2 years. This hospital had a high number of Medicare patients, and it was hit hard by DRGs, the first wave of managed care to hit hospitals. One of my roles was change agent to influence physician practice patterns. We turned around a lot of the cost problems by looking at physician behavior.

The CEO who hired me retired, and a new CEO was brought in. He pulled a group of senior managers together and we went on a two-day retreat. The word was, "You are the group I'm keeping." During my entire tenure, the medical director whom I had been hired to replace never left the premises. The role that he had developed for himself never evolved, and there was no funding for it.

How did it happen?

I was informed that I had been terminated by letter, which the CEO's secretary brought into me about 4:00 one Friday afternoon. This was less than three weeks after the retreat where I was told I was part of the team. This was not too long after I had received a raise, all sorts of commendations, certain financial securities, and parachutes as a reward for a job well done. I was on top of the world, and yet, within no more than four-six weeks, my world came tumbling down. The letter said, "We have one too many physician managers. You've done a good job, but you are the last in and the first out. We can't afford three, and we need two.

I managed to leave the office with my head held high. I thought my world had collapsed. I came home that afternoon and my wife said, "What are you doing home so early?" I never came home at 4:00. I usually came home at 6:00 or 7:00. I sat down on the edge of the chair and I said, "I've lost faith in humanity," and I cried. I don't cry very often, but I cried. To my wife's credit, after a few minutes she picked me up and said, "Go clean up. We're going out, have a dinner, and celebrate the move to the next stage of the rest of our lives."

I forced the CEO to write to the medical staff exactly what had happened. I didn't want to have to explain it to everybody. I knew it would get out, and I wanted the CEO to go up front and explain what happened and why. I also jumped all over him for the way he did it. He needed to have the guts to look me in the eye. I told him I respected the fact that he was paid to make hard decisions. Although I didn't agree with his decision, I respected his right to make that decision. It was just handed to me the wrong way.

What was the worst part of being fired?

The worst part was the abject shock. I knew there were some warning signs—the other fellow never left, a new CEO came in, the CEO and the previous medical director had been friends—and yet I felt fairly secure, mainly because of the rewards I had received, the validation at the retreat, the parachute that was given to me for a job well done. I was still blindsided, and the pain of that time and the pain of the next few days and the humiliation of telling my family and friends was probably the most difficult thing I've ever gone through in my life.

As you look back at your firing, was there a good part to it for your life and for your future?

Yes. It forces you to take stock, use this time to pause and rethink where you are in your career and where you want to be. It validates the fact that you can pick yourself up off the floor and you can wipe the blood off your nose and you can climb up and achieve things that you may not have gotten before through the support of friends and family and network and just digging down deep into yourself. I think the measure of a person is how they respond to adversity. As painful as it is, it tests you. I probably have a greater feeling of self-worth now that I've picked myself up. I had a family that stood by me, a network that stood by me. I had more opportunities than you can shake a stick at. I'm a whole lot smarter. I couldn't say the "f" word for a while. Now I can tell people I was fired. I don't have to tell them I was terminated, or I would explain the situation and not say the word. It is one of those words that sounds like what it is. I think that is called onomatopoeia. "Fired" is a harsh cutting word.

How long did it take to feel better?

I think it took two-four weeks. [We were talking on the phone, and he called to his wife in another room and said, "How long did it take me before I was out of a funk?" She called back, "Four and closer to eight weeks.") For a while, you just beat yourself up.

What helped you?

The first week I called a friend and a professional career counselor whose business it is to counsel and advise people at a time like this. I kept a diary at his recommendation. I wouldn't have done it on my own. I still haven't looked at it. It's here. When we make explicit what was implicit, it has a different meaning. It's like when you are forced to write down your goals and put them on paper, it has a different meaning than if you just think them. The exercise of going through that had a bit of a healing effect, purging yourself of the demons. I recommend that you seek professional advice and don't be too proud to do that and think that you know everything about everything.

I made a business of resurrecting my career and moving forward. Each morning I got dressed, went into the office in my home, and went to work. I kept a calendar, I had hours and I had appointments. I just started turning over stones. Fortunately, I had kept my résumé with most of the physician executive headhunters. I called some key people in the American College of Physician Executives.

I went to work for a consulting firm in three months. That offer had been on the table before. I had copresented with this consulting firm because our hospital was used as a model for how to lower costs by changing physician practice patterns. It always said to me anytime you want to work with us, call us. Plus, I had had the usual bevy of calls we all receive at work, as most of the headhunters are looking for somebody who already has a job, not somebody who doesn't have a job.

Are there things you wish you had or hadn't done?

I've thought about it a 100 million times. At times, I don't think so. I was proud of the job I did. At other times, I've thought I could have been more politically adroit. I could have spent more time with some of the key power players of the hospital.

Are there lessons you have learned?

One of the things I've learned is that we need to take responsibility for all that happens to us. Any time there's failure or something doesn't work out, you have to assume it wasn't all just circumstances. Perhaps there were some things you could have done better, some things you didn't do, or politically you could have been more astute.

Sure there is a political piece to it. The guy in the background came back in and did my job. I was a change agent. I wasn't a caretaker medical director. I had not grown up in that hospital. I didn't have the long history.

Unfortunately, it has made me more skeptical. By nature, I believe in humanity, and I like to have faith and trust in other human beings. This episode has made me a little bit jaded, and I think that is probably wise from a business perspective. I don't like it from a humanitarian perspective, because I tend to believe in the good in people and then they have to prove me wrong. I've become more cynical since then, but I've also come to realize that business is business and if possible try not even to personalize it, because it wasn't personal.

Also, I learned that, as long as you are working for somebody else, there is no absolute security—that no matter what is said or written down there is no absolute security; that changes take place in organizations at lots of different levels all the time; that when you work for someone you are a commodity; and that a lot of times, when a new CEO comes in, he or she makes a lot of changes, right or wrong, good or bad.

Does anything else come to mind?

I've got great things to say about ACPE, because, without the College, I probably never would have gotten some of those positions. I think one of the undervalued parts of the College is the network and the fact that every time I have called anybody and asked for advice and counsel, there was just an outpouring of help from everybody. I don't know if it is underutilized, but I didn't appreciate the power of the organization until I went through that and I'll be forever grateful. That is one of the reasons why I'm so involved and why I'm trying to give back, because I don't know what I would have done without an anchor. I guess I would have survived, but it sure made it a lot easier. We all need anchors in the storm. Word leaked out. People in the College called and said, "Have you considered this? Have you considered that?"

What advice would you give to others in the same situation?

You have to prepare as if it is going to happen. You have to have everything in place as if you could get fired tomorrow. Never, never, never assume that it can't happen to you or that it won't happen to you. If you chronicle most successful business people in life, many of them have had a similar experience somewhere along the way, whether it was in early, middle, or senior management.

Being fired is like being smacked with a whip. You go into your office one day, and, "blam," it happens, and your whole world collapses. Is everything in place? Do you have a network? Do they understand what you do? Is your résumé current? Have you kept yourself in visible positions by writing or speaking or taking leadership roles in the organization? Preparation ahead of time is essential.

Also, take the high road. You don't point fingers. You don't blame what happened on anyone else. In fact, you don't have to blame it on anyone. It's just that certain things happen. You accept your fate. I watched my favorite pro basketball team last night, and they just got shellacked. Some days you just get shellacked, and you just keep your mouth shut and move ahead. Many people get fired, but when you blame other people, you hurt yourself. You're not going to hurt the organization. Sooner or later, it will come back and just kill you.

Second Physician Executive

(At the time of the interview, three months had passed since this physician executive had been fired.)

What position did you have?

I was Vice President for Medical Affairs at a large general hospital.

How did the downsizing happen?

The hospital started eliminating positions over the past two years. It eliminated more than 30 positions, and one of them was the VPMA. Morale was awful. I had been participating in the top management team and selecting people to let go, little realizing that I would be selected. I got 24 hours' notice. The hospital said my firing would be announced the next day. There was a brief discussion, and I said, "l think you are making a mistake."

Can you see any good part it has for you and your career?

There may be. For one thing, I've been in this a long time. Economically, it is no problem, which is fortunate. I can see how someone could really get in difficulty if there is an economic problem.

Did you have a severance package already in place?

Yes. That was in the contract, and I think that is absolutely critical. I wouldn't take a job without it. Basically what is happening is that you essentially work at will. Almost all contracts have a termination clause, so you have to protect yourself. Reductions in force are occurring everywhere. As I talk around, there are a number of VPMAs who have been reduced out of their jobs, so you really have to prepare for it. There is an inherent tension between an administrator and a VPMA, because, as they move into the whole cost versus quality issue, most administrators have no knowledge of quality, but they have the assumption that they know what they are doing. As administrators come under increasing pressure, they resent physicians in general and firing them makes a nice scapegoating. These things are going to probably get worse. I think traditional administrators are going to be replaced by physician administrators. So there is more hostility and attempts to get them out of the environment.

Did you feel the initial numbness of shock and devastation or, because you had a good severance package, did you pretty much take it in stride?

Well, it really knocks you back on your feet, whether you have a severance package or not.

How long did it take you to regain your equilibrium, or have you?

I think I've pretty well gained that. I got a lot of support. I got support, surprisingly, from the medical staff, even from people with whom I had raised major issues. That support was pleasant and surprising. I've had support from my family. Also from other physicians in ACPE. People called me, and I called them. I started to network. I'm going out tomorrow to look into some sort of thing in terms of consulting.

What helped?

The announcement appeared in the newspaper the next day. A subspecialist called me up and said he wanted to work out a position for me. He thought I had talent that would be useful in putting together an organization.

Are there lessons you have learned?

One of the key things that I see was that I was recruited in by an administrator who subsequently left. When there is a change of administrators, there is a time of testing. That person coming in has little knowledge of what you have done and may have a preconceived picture of the position. The person may well have had problems with physicians in the past and bring those prejudices to bear on you.

Do you have any advice to others?

Yes. It is devastating to get fired. You probably ought to sit back and look at what you want to do in the future. Then start to network with people. I started networking right away. I set up a home office, put in a fax machine.

It is very important to have support early on. I didn't want to move geographically, so that immediately limited my choices. But I'm a very senior person. I wouldn't have kept working too much longer anyhow. I've talked to other people who are much younger, and it took them up to a year to find something. It's a different situation for me, because I'm not looking for that sort of thing. It's important to talk to people you have worked with in the past in other management positions and try to establish a connection there.

It is absolutely critical to get a good attorney, particularly if you can get someone who is knowledgeable about hospitals. If you are older, the firing organization will try to say that you are retired, but it is important to get it to say in any agreement that it was a reduction of force, not retirement, because then a restrictive covenant doesn't hold. If you are recruited into a hospital, most contracts say you can't take another similar position within so many miles within a year or two after you quit. That would hold if you retired. As a result of using an attorney, I was able to negotiate very favorable terms. That's important, on top of whatever sort of parachute you have. I had a couple of months to work this out.

How did you hear about that person?

I talked to an attorney that I had worked with and asked who would you recommend?

Conclusion

Firing seems like a devastating event, even if recruiters call you fairly regularly about other possibilities. The rejection feels personal, and it takes some time to get over the initial shock. The support of a well-developed network of professional contacts, family, and friends softens the blow. After a short period of grieving, it is important to get busy and contact people in order to move to the next phase of your career.

References

1. Tiffan, W. "When Downsizing Points to You." Presentation at ACPE Perspectives in Medical Management, Chicago, Ill., May 1995.
2. Baber, A., and Waymon, L. *How to Fireproof Your Career. Survival Strategies for Volatile Times*. New York, N.Y.: Berkley Books, 1995.
3. *Ibid.*, p. 80.
4. *Ibid.*, pp. 77-9.

Chapter Twelve

Helpful Tools for the Job Search—Ways to Keep Your Sanity

In Chapter 11, a physician executive mentioned the benefits of keeping a journal if you are fired. A journal can be a useful tool throughout the job search. You can keep track of the daily tasks necessary to pursue a new position, give concrete formation to your goals, and change the thoughts in your head from negative to positive to keep an essential optimistic outlook for finding a job. Keeping a journal can also help you cope with the stresses of your present job. Many have reported that the reflective time required by writing helps them to make sense of and find meaning in their lives.

Journal

I suggest that you write in a journal 10 minutes a day, 5 days week. A journal is whatever kind of paper you like. I like wide-ruled, thick, five-subject spiral notebooks with white paper and blue lines. Maybe you like yellow legal paper, although most doctors I know don't. You can type on your word processor if that suits you better. I write with cheap pens of which I have an unlimited supply. When I've used an expensive pen, I spend all my time worrying about when I'll lose the pen rather than thinking about what I am writing. If you like an expensive pen, buy one, buy two. The point is—be specific about your likes and dislikes and pamper yourself as much as possible. Write in your favorite spot with all the utensils, accompaniments, and frills that please you. Cater to your slightest whim. You don't need to discipline yourself about what materials you use or where you write. A large part of getting yourself to write in a journal is getting over whatever kind of discipline or even abuse you suffered at the hand of some teacher during your education process. If ever your paper was snatched from you and read to the whole class, you probably have significant paralysis to overcome.

In this journal that you have carefully chosen, do a special kind of writing called freewriting. When you freewrite, you write whatever comes into your mind. You don't worry about spelling, punctuation, grammar, or anything that some English teacher told you to always worry about. "There are no fixed rules for journal writing....It's not a place to condemn nor judge, but a place to observe. Pay no attention at all to your 'style' of writing."[1] Your handwriting or typing does not have to be neat or accurate. No one will see anything you write. There is only one catch. For the process to work well, you need to keep writing until the 10 minutes are up. Set a timer if you have to. I know that two pages of nonstop writing in my spiral notebook always equals ten minutes. If you can't think of anything to write, just say over and over, " I can't think of anything to write. I can't think of anything to write. I wonder when I will think of something." But keep moving your pen and writing something, even if it is nonsense. There is a reason for this. Ideas will pop into your head if you keep writing that won't come if you just sit thinking.

Keep this freewriting private. If you momentarily hate your boss, it's good to write about it. It is not good for him or her to see it. If you write something that would be especially dangerous for someone to see, tear it up when you finish. You'll probably discover that writing takes you places you didn't know you were going to go. You'll begin writing about one idea, and then, suddenly, some other thought pops into your head. Write it down. Don't discipline yourself to stay on a particular subject. Your very best ideas may come trailing after the strangest thoughts.

Marion describes the journal specifically for the pursuit of a job: "Your career search journal is an important way to track your physical and emotional progress, to hear what you have to say to yourself. Record doubts, ideas, impressions, anything interesting that happened that you might want to remember."[2] Leider describes it in broader terms: "When you write in a journal, you're not composing an essay, only recording the unedited expressions of your inner experience. You write in it day by day as much as possible to keep yourself in an ongoing relationship with whatever is taking place inside yourself....Journaling helps you observe your inner conversation more objectively....A journal is a mirror. It's a good listener, a tool for self-guidance, a road map of growth....Some never go back to read in their journals. Others reread continuously to get a feeling of trends in their life."[3] You decide which is helpful for you.

As I have mentioned, I am the spouse of a physician executive. A journal can be beneficial to the spouse as well as to the physician executives. I keep a journal except when I forget to. I can forget for a month at a time. Even though I teach the concept and know it is helpful, I still have lapses of not doing it. I want you to know I know how difficult it will be to get yourself to do this. However, it is worth the effort.

We have made two geographic moves. I did not want to make the first move. I did want to make the second one, but the stresses of moving were great, even though I felt I was going home again. Following is a journal entry during the stressful time of moving. I let you see movies of my mind to see how incoherent, rambling, and confusing a journal entry can be.

Sample of journal entry during a job change and move

Friday I am doing a program in Cape Cod. I speak from 8-12 with an hour for lunch and then speak from 1-4. At noon someone hands me a note saying—They are having trouble with your house closing. Adrenaline rushes. I call the law office. Earlier in the week we had signed a power of attorney to a lawyer so he could do the closing for us. He had transferred the money we were borrowing from the bank to the closing destination. However, I did not remember and the realtor did not remind me to transfer the cash money from the sale of our Orlando house to the closing. Mercifully I had wired that money to a NC bank. I didn't have phone numbers of the 2 people from the NC bank that had processed our loan and had opened the account where that money sat. With 4 phone calls it was worked out but once again I am trying to calm myself.

Use a journal to write goals

Dr. Lee Pulos did research that showed only 4 percent of the population write down their goals. However, those who do write down their goals achieve them almost 100 percent of the time.[4] "You need to have a clear picture of what you want with no inner conflict about whether you deserve it or not."[5] "To be successful you have to believe that you deserve success. You have to have an image of yourself so tangible that you can reach out and touch it."[6]

Writing in your journal is a way to make the goal tangible. If you write out a goal, your brain thinks it, your hand writes it, your eyes see it clearly on the paper, and your subconscious and the universe plan ways to make it happen. "Setting down your plans on paper takes you a step further than just deciding on a career goal and talking about it with others. It constitutes a deeper commitment to yourself. Also, seeing it on paper makes it more concrete."[7] If you keep your goals where you can see them each day, you can determine if you are truly spending your time trying to accomplish them or if you value other things more. If the latter, be honest with yourself and change your goals.

If I am overwhelmed with too many tasks and think I'm a bit off track, I will pick up my journal and write the answers to these questions:

- Is this what I want to be doing?
- Does this move me toward my goal?
- What is that nagging irritation?
- Can I do anything about it now? If not, I write it down so I don't use energy trying to remember it or trying to forget it. I can deal with it later and get back to working on my goal.

Make a list of your goals—things you want to do or accomplish. Make it long, imaginative, demanding of yourself. "One of the most interesting immediate results of writing your goals down clearly, concisely, and without ambiguity, and then memorizing them, is that you will feel better when you have done so.

The reason for this is that...you are doing something your biocomputer has been wanting you to do. It is as though the biocomputer heaves a great sigh of relief and says, 'At last. Now I know where we are going.'"[8]

Self-Talk

A journal is also a place to observe your self-talk—the kind of thinking that goes on in your head all day long. If you see what self-talk is going on in your head, you can change it. "People who are optimistic tend to find jobs faster. They have more energy and follow up on leads. They tell themselves positive things."[9] "If you fail to control your own thoughts, you will have difficulty controlling anything else."[10] "Charles Garfield, in his book *Peak Performers*...suggests that if you can visualize a positive outcome and say self-assuring things to yourself, you greatly increase the chances of reaching your goal."[11] While writing, you see your own negative self-talk and empty it onto the page. Then you can replace it with positive thoughts.

When you write a negative thought, you'll know that's the program your brain computer is running. You have to install a different program using a quite specific method. The new program can be a positive thought about behavior or a picture in your head of a goal you want to achieve. "If you want the new program to be a permanent part of your subconscious, you have to repeat it to yourself under two very specific conditions, 12-15 times a day for 14 or more days (i.e., about 200 repetitions.)[12] The more the better. Every time the negative program starts in your head, substitute the new one. That worry and negative thought can be a reminder to do the repetitions.

"If you trigger a relaxation response before you do the rehearsal, the new positive thoughts tend to be absorbed much more quickly."[13] "If you become exhausted, highly emotional, or under the influence of alcohol or other drugs and the old stimulus occurs, the brain may very well go to the old response. You can't do anything about that, except try not to be in those situations. The more you rehearse, the less likely a reversion is, but the old program is always there and may play from time to time."[14]

Leider describes this process as visualization. "Visualization means talking to yourself silently in a soft but firm tone....Deep prayer, biofeedback, meditation, positive thinking all begin with visualization. It's all a matter of getting yourself into a receptive state."[15] Peter Senge, in *The Fifth Discipline*, describes how some form of meditation helps people excel. "[P]eople committed to continually developing personal mastery practice some form of 'meditation.' Whether it is through contemplative prayer or other methods of simply 'quieting' the conscious mind, regular meditative practice can be extremely helpful in working more productively with the subconscious mind....In our normal highly active state of mind, the subconscious is deluged with a welter of contradictory thoughts and feelings. In a quieter state of mind, when we focus on something of particular importance, some aspect of our vision, the subconscious is undistracted....[D]uring that time) people with high levels of personal mastery direct their focus....[T]hey focus on the desired result itself, not the 'process' or the means they assume necessary to achieve that result."[16]

"Since visualizations only have a life-span of about 36 hours, you'll need to repeat this process daily, until you've truly changed your behavior or reached your goal."[17] "[S]etting aside time for visualizations each day is like an artist's brushstroke toward the completion of the painting."[18]

Dr. Lee Pulos claims we say between 45,000 and 51,000 words to ourselves each day.[4] Only an experienced mediator can go for 11 seconds without self-talk. For a lot of people, much of what they are saying to themselves has a doomsday theme to it.

"You participate in a daily dialogue—everything you say to yourself and others during the day—all thoughts both deliberate and spontaneous. Your dialogue is so important because it is the way you give instructions to yourself—both to your body and to your mind. It is important to change your dialogue to yourself and others from negative, self-destructive things to positive self-enhancing things.

"You are what you tell yourself you are. You feel what you tell yourself you feel. You become what you tell yourself. It doesn't matter whether or not you actually believe the new dialogue. In fact, it will not be true in the beginning, and it will feel strange and uncomfortable. The essence of change is to do something enough until it becomes true."[19]

The repetition of positive statements may strike you as contrived and too easy. If you try it, you'll find it takes quite a bit of discipline to control the thoughts in your head, but it can be done. You may think your positive statement is a lie. That doesn't matter—say it to yourself anyway. It will become the truth.

The use of a journal and positive self-talk will spur you on to do the work necessary to find your next job and enhance your career.

References

1. Leider, R. *Life Skills*. San Diego, Calif.: Pfeiffer & Company, 1994, p. 184.
2. Marion, P. *Crisis Proof Your Career.* New York, N.Y.: Berkley Books, 1994, p. 172.
3. Leider, R., *op cit.,* pp. 183-4.
4. Pulos, L.. *The Power of Visualization.* An audiotape series produced by Nightingale-Conant Corporation, 7300 N. Lehigh Ave., Niles, Ill. 60714, 800/323-5552.
5. Marion, P. *op. cit.,* p. 31.

6. *Ibid.*, p. 97.

7. *Ibid.*, p. 141.

8. Thomas, P. *Advanced Psycho-Cybernetics.* New York, N.Y.: Perigee Books, 1992, p. 128.

9. Marion, P., *op. cit.*, p. 33.

10. Thomas, P., *op. cit.*, p. 182.

11. Marion, P., *op. cit.*, p. 78.

12. Dwyer, C. *The Shifting Sources of Power and Influence.* Tampa, Fla.: American College of Physician Executives, 1991, p. 52.

13. Dwyer, C., *op. cit.*, p. 53.

14. *Ibid.*, p. 55.

15. Leider, R., *op. cit.*, p. 180.

16. Senge, P. *The Fifth Discipline.* New York, N.Y.: Doubleday Currency, 1990, p. 164.

17. Leider, R., *op. cit.*, p. 183.

18. Marion, P., *op. cit.*, p. 119.

19. Covington, F., and Seagrave, A. *CHAANGE Handbook.* Charlotte, N.C.: CHAANGE, 1986, p.9.

Other Reading

Alexander, J. *Dare to Change.* New York, N.Y.: A Signet Book, New American Library, 1984.

Baber, A., and Waymon, L. *How to Fireproof Your Career. Survival Strategies for Volatile Times.* New York, N.Y.: Berkley Books, 1995.

Covey, S. *The 7 Habits of Highly Effective People.* New York, N.Y.: Simon and Schuster, 1989.

Elbow, Peter. *Writing Without Teachers.* London, England: Oxford University Press, 1973.

Gillett, R. *Change Your Mind. Change Your World.* New York, N.Y.: Simon and Schuster, 1992.

Wallen, E. "Job Pressures Seen Fueling Rise in Doctors' Stress Levels." *Physicians Financial News*, Oct. 15, 1993, pp. 15-6.

Wheelis, A. *How People Change.* New York, N.Y.: Harper Colophon Books, 1973.